# Everyday Yoga

# Everyday
# Yoga

## At-Home Routines to Enhance Fitness, Build Strength, and Restore Your Body

### Sage Rountree

VELO.

Boulder, Colorado

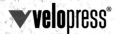

3002 Sterling Circle, Suite 100
Boulder, Colorado 80301-2338 USA
(303) 440-0601  Fax (303) 444-6788
E-mail velopress@competitorgroup.com

Distributed in the United States and Canada by Ingram Publisher Services

A Cataloging-in-Publication record for this book is available from the Library of Congress.
ISBN 978-1-937715-35-9

For information about purchasing VeloPress books,
please call (800) 811-4210, ext. 2138, or visit www.velopress.com.

Photographs by Seth K. Hughes
Cover design by Brenda Gallagher
Interior design by Vicki Hopewell

15  16  17 / 10  9  8  7  6  5  4  3  2  1

To Wanda and Roy Williams

# contents

## 3

### everyday yoga practices

## 4

### organizing your everyday yoga

**If you can breathe, you can do yoga.** | Because yoga means union—connection of your awareness to what is happening *right now*— you don't have to lift a finger to do it. This may come as a relief to those of you who quake at the idea of bending a knee into lotus pose (which isn't depicted in this book) or twisting arms into a full bind (that isn't, either). But practicing a little bit of yoga most days, whether through poses, meditation, or breathing, will vastly improve the experience you have in your body and mind.

Everyday yoga is just that—yoga that's accessible and that's meant to be done daily to help you feel happier and healthier. In this book, you'll learn routines and practices that will build strength in your core, flexibility in your hips, relaxation in your body, and focus in your mind. Practicing yoga will enhance whatever else you do, be it a sports competition, parenting, running errands, or simply being in your body.

Part 1 introduces a menu approach to building your everyday yoga practice. I'll explain how to create everything from a simple "snack" (a short routine of a few poses that lasts only a few minutes) to a full "meal" (a long routine of several poses plus breath exercises and meditation that lasts more than an hour). You'll also learn commonsense guidelines for a safe yoga practice, including an easy formula for helping you choose a balanced set of poses and routines.

"Everyday yoga is just that—yoga that's accessible and meant to be done daily."

Part 2 explains, through beautiful photographs and clear directions, how to complete a selection of well-balanced routines that will help establish and evolve your daily practice. Because these offerings are both balanced and simple, you'll feel nourished by following just one routine per day. This daily practice will help keep you injury-free and feeling strong in your other physical endeavors.

Part 3 suggests ways to combine the poses and routines from Part 2 into short and long practices. You'll find practices to build strength, improve balance, and increase flexibility, as well as to help you unwind and improve focus. Part 4 provides sample weekly and monthly plans to help you determine the right frequency and intensity of your everyday practice.

As you grow comfortable with this approach and build your repertoire, you can riff on the routines to suit your fitness level, body type, time commitment, personality, and appetite. Cues in the routines will help you stablish your exertion level and appetite, whether it's for something

**"**Riff on the routines to suit your fitness level, body type . . . and appetite. . . . You will build a stronger, more flexible, injury-resistant body."

spicy, sweet, or with a little seasoning. For example, some days you might have a hunger for spicier standing poses and backbends; other days you may want to settle into sweeter, more relaxing poses like restorative folds and twists. Following one routine will help you feel satisfied and relaxed; through enjoying several, by practicing either the à la carte options in Part 2 or one of the full-practice options in Part 3, you will build a stronger, more flexible, injury-resistant body.

Just as learning to cook gives you the tools to nourish yourself, learning to practice yoga at home gives you the tools to feed your soul, enhance fitness, and live healthfully. Yoga doesn't have to happen in a studio, and you don't have to take 60 or 90 minutes to complete a routine that will leave you feeling balanced, centered, strong, and calm. The tools to do yoga yourself, every day, are right here in your hands, in your body, and in your breath.

# building your
## everyday
# practice

# how to
# **use this book**

This is not a how-to book (for that, you should study in person with an experienced teacher). This is a what-to book, designed to inspire you to practice yoga every day and to create routines that nourish you.

Sitting down to a meal gives you an opportunity to do more than just feed yourself. Eating can engage the senses—taste, of course, but also smell, touch, sight, and even sound—and thus put you more fully in the present. Whether you are eating alone or communing with friends, dining gives you a chance to connect completely to what is happening in the moment. The same goes for practicing yoga, which is why I chose a menu approach for this book.

## Using the Routines and Practices

The routines in Part 2 are a visual guide to creating your everyday practice, with some instruction. Part 3 demonstrates how to pick from the menu of options in Part 2 to create short and long practices. Some days you'll want only one routine; other days you'll crave more. Balance comes when you alternate between short and long practices, giving your body what it needs from moment to moment.

**"**This is a what-to book, designed to inspire you to practice yoga every day and to create routines that nourish you."

If you are a visual learner, you'll probably do best referring to the pictures. If you are a verbal learner, use the text directions; you can supplement those shorthand cues by referring to my books *The Athlete's Guide to Yoga* and *The Runner's Guide to Yoga*. If you are a kinesthetic learner, you might like the video renditions of these poses, available at sagerountree.com/everydayyoga.

## Seasoning to Taste

The routines in Part 2 include modification cues to make a pose sweeter or spicier or to season to taste. I use these terms instead of denoting levels or stages of the pose, because how you do yoga best is dependent completely on you, not on any external ideal of a pose or an exercise (see options below). Choosing the sweeter variation of a pose will generally require less effort and yield less intensity; going spicier will heat things up and add intensity. In some cases, variations are just that—different flavors, not degrees of intensity—so you'll see cues to season poses differently.

| **SPICIER** | **SWEETER** | **SEASONING** |
|---|---|---|
| To up the challenge a notch, choose the spicier variation. | Find greater ease with the sweeter modification cues. | Seasoning cues yield a result that can be spicy or sweet, depending on your body. |

**"**Make a pose sweeter or spicier, or season to taste."

Depending on your own experience and physical make-up, what feels spicy to me may be mild to you; simply think of these modification cues as giving your practice a palette of choices.

## Pacing, Breath, and Movement

As you adjust the seasoning in each routine according to your taste, you might also choose to modify by pulsing dynamically from pose to pose several times before holding in a pose for several breaths or by flowing back and forth between poses. How many times you flow and how long you hold each pose is up to you. Five to 10 breaths is a rough range for flowing, while 10 to 25 breaths is a rough range for holding. In challenging poses, you might like or need to move along more quickly to the next pose; in relaxing poses, you might like to stay longer. If you choose a modified approach to the routines in this book, then take the breath cues as a suggestion. You can experiment to determine what works best for your breath and body. To make a routine spicier, you might pulse from pose to pose several times before holding in a particular pose for several breaths; to make a routine sweeter, you might pulse only once or twice before holding.

Generally, when you move dynamically, inhale as you lift, and exhale as you lower. For pulses where part of the movement is more challenging, exhale as you execute the challenging movement. This helps engage your core muscles to support and stabilize the pelvis and spine. Listen to your body and your breath, and you'll find the best approach to every move.

**"**Yoga is a system for connection, and the poses are just one entry point to this union. Breath is another."

Finally, yoga is far more than simply making shapes in space. Yoga is a system for connection, and the poses are just one entry point to this union. Breath is another, as is meditation. Part 2 concludes with some very simple breath and mindfulness exercises. Combine these with the physical routines, and you'll be on your way to well-rounded, whole-being health.

# guidelines
## for practicing yoga

As you begin with a customized approach to building your home practice, it's important to review the building blocks and establish good yoga habits. The guidelines outlined here will help you develop and transform your home yoga practice. Being smart and safe allows you to create and practice routines that build overall fitness, satisfy your appetite, and leave you feeling content.

## Alignment

To learn good alignment in each of the poses, read books, watch instructional videos, take introductory-level classes at a local studio, or book one-on-one lessons with an experienced yoga teacher in your area. The style of yoga that you study during in-person classes will inform your knowledge of poses, including the general rules of alignment for their various expressions. Ultimately, you'll need to figure out the best alignment in your own body, and home practice can help you discover it.

**Remember mountain pose** I The routines in this book generally start with a home-base pose like mountain pose (standing tall) or table pose

**"**Being smart and safe allows you to create and practice routines that build overall fitness, satisfy your appetite, and leave you feeling content."

(on hands and knees). Before you move your body into any other shape, remember the principles of good alignment in mountain pose: level pelvis, long spine, relaxed upper body. They will inform every pose you do—and good alignment will protect your spine and hips.

**Long spine** | Although the routines in this book explicitly focus on taking the spine through a full range of motion, you'll do well to protect your spine from extreme movement at any one point. In general, you want to distribute movement across the joints of the spine. This is especially true during backbends and inversions. Aim to keep the lumbar curve in your low back from doing all the work, and don't let the cervical curve in your neck crane too much, either. A helpful way to remember this is to cue "long spine" to yourself as you come into a pose. This cue will help you to protect your neck in backbends and inversions and to evenly distribute the work in your spine when doing backbends, forward folds, side bends, and twists.

**Knees and toes agree** | Sometimes you'll be pointing your feet in the same direction, and sometimes you'll be pointing one or both feet away from anatomical neutral. When your feet don't point in the same direction, be sure that you originate the action from the hip, not the feet, so that your knee points in the same direction as your toes.

## Equipment

Start with the right equipment. A sharp high-quality knife, a few pieces of good cookware, and top-quality salt and olive oil can be used to better effect than a kitchen full of dull blades, warped pans, and obscure specialty products. In the same way, as you buy yoga equipment, favor quality and versatility over quantity and specialized function.

**Yoga mat** | Typically considered an essential piece of yoga equipment, a yoga mat provides cushion and traction and helps define space for your practice. The market is full of options, from thin and lightweight to thick and heavy. If you can, test your options at a local outfitter or yoga studio. If your practice will involve a lot of time in supine or prone poses, a thicker, spongier mat may suit you (I like the prAna ECO Pro line for mat practices). For standing and more dynamic routines, a thinner or harder mat can offer better grip (I like the Manduka Pro line for standing practices).

A mat is not required for home practice. Standing poses can be done on the floor, either barefoot or in shoes, and low-to-the-ground routines can be done on carpet or grass, maybe with a beach towel to cushion you. If you wear socks when practicing on carpet or a hard surface, consider socks with no-slip bottoms.

**Yoga blocks** | Blocks help you develop flexibility by bringing the floor closer to your hands in standing poses and providing added support during mat work. Choose a block that is firm but that has a little give to it, ideally one made of heavy foam or cork. You can find yoga blocks at health food and big-box stores, as well as online (the blocks used in this book are from huggermugger.com). Buy two while you're at it.

**Yoga strap** | This is a useful tool for developing your flexibility. Buy an 8- or 10-foot woven strap with a metal D-ring or plastic buckle, or make a provisional strap from a necktie, belt, or woven dog leash.

**Clothes** | For everyday yoga practice, you don't need any special clothes. Choose pants or shorts that don't constrict your movement. Tuck in your shirt, or choose a shirt tight enough that you won't have a mouthful of fabric when you're upside down.

## Know Your Limits

Although your growth and progress in yoga can depend on pushing through perceived boundaries, the challenge is often more subtle: to do less and relax more. Despite what you might be used to in sports training, you should not experience pain when you practice. Be particularly wary of sharp discomfort at a joint. Depending on the routines you do, you may register effort in your muscles as you challenge your strength or as you stretch and near the limits of your flexibility. Just as cooks can watch a thermometer to avoid overcooking or burning food, you have your breath to help you gauge the heat you build in your body while you practice and to help you know when to lessen the intensity.

**Effort and ease** | Seek to find a healthy balance between working enough and working too much. To keep your yoga diet balanced, be sure you aren't developing too much of a sweet tooth—cleaving only to the easy routines—and, conversely, that you aren't overloading on spice at every meal. If you find yourself sweating, grunting, and powering

**"** Seek to find a healthy balance between working enough and working too much."

through poses that challenge you, more ease is in order. Conversely, if you tend to always keep things easy, consider upping the challenge. Use the sweet and spicy and seasoning cues to help you strike a good balance of effort and ease, stress and rest, over the course of your days, weeks, and months.

## Balance Is Key: The 6-4-2 Principle

Seek balance in your body, because balance is the key to preventing injury. An acute injury is the result of a fall or force imbalance. An overuse injury is the result of some imbalance in the body—front to back, left to right, top to bottom. An imbalance between stress and rest can result in injury and create mood problems that can affect your practice. An everyday yoga practice will help you go a long way toward finding and keeping balance in your body, mind, and spirit. As your practice grows, you'll learn to intuit what you need for balance. Some days, it may be more or targeted work; other days, it will be rest or meditation.

Just as your goal is to eat a balanced diet, the goal of your everyday yoga should be to find balance in your practice and overall health. Your home practice should generally follow the simple rules of the 6-4-2 principle:

- Include poses that move your spine in **6** directions.
- Target your hips in **4** areas.
- Challenge your core in **2** ways.

**Balanced spine** | Your spine is capable of moving forward and back (flexion and extension), from side to side (lateral flexion in both directions), and round and round (twisting in both directions). If, over the course of the day, you spend much of your time sitting—or worse, if you spend that seated time on the bike saddle, in your car seat, or slouching at your desk—you're encouraging flexion but missing out on the other ways your spine can move. Practicing yoga poses can really help, because the poses will move you out of the plane of forward motion and into side bending, twisting, and backward bending. This helps balance strength and flexibility in the muscles that support your spine—reducing back pain, improving posture, and generally making you feel good.

**Balanced hips** | The hips and thighs power your movement through space. As with the muscles that support the spine, the muscles that power the hips are usually focused on moving you forward. If you spend a lot of your day sitting in a chair or engage in an exercise that features repetitive movements, like most sports, it's easy to develop an imbalance between tightness in the front of the hip (the hip flexors) and weakness in the back (the glutes), as well as between the inner lines of the thighs (adductors) and the outer hips (abductors). To cultivate balance and prevent injury, focus on the four lines of the hip: front, back, inside, and outside. All the routines in Part 2 include work in each of these areas.

**Balanced core** | Your core supports your spine as you move it in articulation or stabilization. *Articulation* means you're moving through the joints between each segment of the spine. *Stabilization* means you're engaging your core muscles to hold your spine steady in space. To maintain good

**"**Creating a balanced practice sequence is similar to preparing a balanced meal."

posture and keep your spine well supported, include both articulation exercises (e.g., cat/cow poses) and stabilization exercises (e.g., plank poses) in your home practice.

## Balance in Orientation

How you combine the routines in this book can help you achieve balance in your everyday practice. Creating a balanced practice sequence is similar to preparing a balanced meal. In general, select a mix of routines that allow you to spend some time doing the following:

* Lying on your back, facing up, as well as lying on your belly or on hands and knees, facing down
* Sitting and standing
* Facing the short edge of your mat, as well as facing the long edge of your mat

These simple guidelines will encourage you to move your body in various orientations to gravity, which builds better balance and awareness of your body in space. If you are following the 6-4-2 principle (discussed earlier), you are naturally moving your spine in every direction and encouraging better balance by periodically changing your orientation on the mat.

# creating
# nourishing practices

A balanced food diet is based on macronutrients (carbohydrates, protein, and fats) and micronutrients (vitamins, minerals, and trace elements), and you also need regular intake of water to survive. Similarly, a balanced physical yoga diet will include several key features, a variety of lesser ingredients, and your breath.

## Macronutrients

A balanced physical yoga diet includes the following:

* Moving the spine in every direction available to it: forward, backward, from side to side, and twisting in both directions
* Addressing the hips from every angle: front, back, inside, and outside
* Challenging the muscles to articulate the vertebrae in the spine, as well as to stabilize the core

Consistently eating an imbalanced food diet can lead to health problems; consistently neglecting a path of physical movement can do the same. If your yoga practice focuses on forward folding, but no backward bending, and you already spend much of your day sitting, you'll be amplifying an imbalance instead of correcting it. For this reason, you should remember the 6-4-2 principle discussed earlier. Applying it will help you keep your yoga routines nutritionally well balanced.

The amount of macronutrients and micronutrients that you take in over the course of a week is far more important than what you eat during any given meal. If you have no protein at breakfast, you can make it up at lunch. If you don't eat many carbohydrates at lunch, you can add some in at supper. The same holds true for your yoga practice. If you include a balanced physical yoga diet over the course of each week, you don't necessarily need every individual routine or practice to be balanced. Instead, you can pick and choose from a menu of options based on what's available—the space you have, the time you have, even what you happen to be wearing—and address any imbalances in the next practice, in a targeted yoga snack, or during the rest of the week.

## Micronutrients

The full spectrum of micronutrients, although important to your overall health, is not something you have to consume at every meal. This same principle applies to your balanced yoga diet. Although side bending is good for you, that doesn't mean that gate pose must be part of every yoga practice; just aim to include side bending, whether it's with gate pose or some alternative shape, over the course of your yoga week. Long-term neglect of movements of your body can cause you to accrue an imbalance of micronutrients or to develop health problems.

## Water

You can survive for several days without food, but lacking water is a more dire issue. To continue our analogy, breath is like water—without it, you won't be around for long. Don't forget to drink in long, deep breaths during your yoga practice. The more attention you give to your breath, the more subtleties you'll find in its movement and timing. In this way, your experience of your breath can be like savoring a complex wine. It changes over time and in different contexts; its flavors can complement or clash with what the body is doing in the moment.

## Satisfy Your Appetite

With the concept of macronutrients, micronutrients, and water in mind, choose your yoga practices according to your hunger, taste, and thirst. Maybe you have only a little time to dedicate to yoga in a day and you have a hankering for backward bending; choose a routine with more backward bends. Maybe you want a quick routine to do in bed or on the floor; choose a supine six-moves-of-the-spine practice. Or maybe you're hungry for a feast; choose or create a longer, multiroutine practice like those in Part 3. Some days all you need is a long drink of water; in that case, get comfortable and enjoy one of the breath practices presented in Part 2.

Some poses may hold less appeal for you. In that case, a little reverse engineering can help you find an appropriate substitute. First, consider

**"**Drink in long, deep breaths during your yoga practice. The more attention you give to your breath, the more subtleties you'll find in its movement and timing."

the intention of the pose: Is it a forward fold? A backbend? Does it target a particular body part? Next, look for an alternative. Sometimes simply changing a pose's relationship to gravity will make it more palatable. Instead of downward-facing dog, for example, give the pose a quarter-turn and try downward-facing dog with your hands on the wall. Instead of lizard lunge, flip the pose over into half happy baby.

Worse, certain poses might not agree with your constitution. Perhaps you feel sharp pain or discomfort when you move into the poses, or you find yourself holding your breath or breathing very shallowly. Avoid such poses; consult with an experienced teacher or a physical therapist to address the root of the problem.

# where, when, and how often to **practice**

## Where to Practice

This book is your tool to a nourishing home practice. Don't grow so reliant on studio classes that you miss out on the bread and butter of yoga: your home practice. However, you can keep your practice fresh by checking in periodically with teachers, whether in drop-in classes, workshops, or private lessons. You'll get the power of practicing with a group, as well as a teacher's eyes on your alignment. When you practice regularly at home, you may develop habits that could become harmful over time; having a teacher assess your form will keep you safe, and learning new routines or approaches will keep you inspired.

Once you feel comfortable with your everyday yoga practice, visiting new teachers or studios can be like trying ethnic cuisines or a new restaurant. Different yoga styles will have a different seasoning profile. Some are heavy on inversions; some are heavy on props. Some use a liberal dash of chanting; some sprinkle philosophy throughout. Venturing beyond your routine from time to time will keep up your appetite for yoga, and you may find yourself riffing on these new flavors on your mat at home.

If you have the room, set up a dedicated space for yoga at home or work. Ideally, this space will be free of distractions, such as pets or children wandering through, as well as free of computer and device screens. If such a space is unavailable, mute your phone and work to sustain your focus on your body and breath. The better you get at practicing in the face of distractions and interruptions, the better you'll be at maintaining concentration in any situation.

## When to Practice

Practice at a time of day that suits your taste. If you have time and inclination in the morning, include a warm-up and a standing routine. Standing poses also make a good mid-afternoon snack or pre-workout dynamic warm-up (in that case, opt to flow from pose to pose rather than holding poses statically). At the end of your workout, include a core-focused mat routine. After a day at work, try a warm-up followed by a mat routine for a grounding practice. Enjoy a closing sequence to help you unwind before bed. Because the routines outlined in Part 2 are bite-sized, you can pick and choose what works for you no matter the time of day.

## How Often to Practice

Although this book is called *Everyday Yoga*, you don't need to practice every day to see results. Including a routine or two every other day, or even two or three times a week, will have a big positive effect on your mental and physical health and well-being. Part 4 offers sample yoga schedules to get you started.

# everyday yoga
# routines

These routines will help you develop a menu approach to your home practice. If you are an athlete, you can include warm-ups before a workout to loosen your body and elevate your heart rate. Afterward, standing poses will build stability and mat work will help you strengthen your core and maintain balance in your hips. The cool-down routines help complete a longer practice or work well as stand alone routines to speed recovery or relaxation practices. Throughout, you'll see cues to make poses sweeter, spicier, or differently seasoned. Use these as starting points for customizing your practice to transform and restore your body.

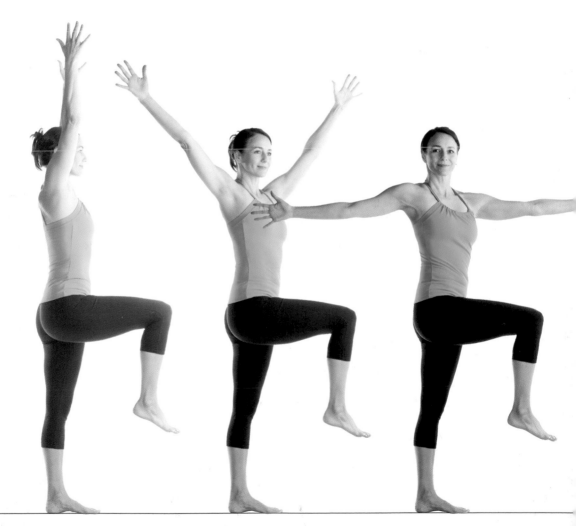

spicier | sweeter | seasoning

# whole-body warm-ups | Use warm-up sequences as stand-alone yoga snacks, or string several together to make a gentle practice. These also work well as dynamic warm-up routines before your workout.

## standing six moves of the spine

*A perfect break from time at your desk. No mat needed!*

Stand in mountain pose. Bend your knees slightly and rest hands on thighs.

Inhale and lift your tailbone, chest, and gaze for standing cow; exhale and round your back for standing cat. Repeat for several rounds.

From mountain pose, inhale and bring your arms overhead; exhale and side bend to the left. Hold for several breaths. Switch sides.

From mountain pose, inhale and bring your arms overhead; exhale and side twist to the right, bending your left knee for standing twist. Hold for a stretch, or build core strength by pulsing the twist from side to side. Switch sides. ● *Spicier: Side twist and keep your hips facing forward, twisting only from the waist upward.* ● *Spicier: Side twist to the right, bend your right knee, and lift it to hip height, keeping hips and knees facing forward.*

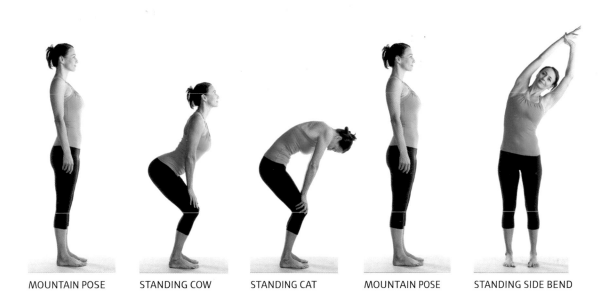

MOUNTAIN POSE          STANDING COW          STANDING CAT          MOUNTAIN POSE          STANDING SIDE BEND

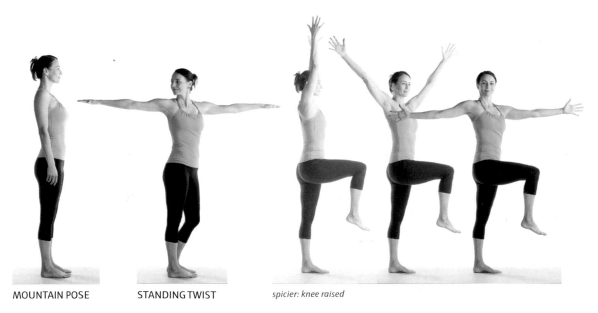

MOUNTAIN POSE          STANDING TWIST          *spicier: knee raised*

## six moves of the spine, kneeling

*This works well from kneeling, with the added benefit of stretching tight quadriceps and ankles, but if you find yourself chair-bound, like on a trip, try this sequence right in your seat.*

Sit on your heels and rest your hands on your thighs. Inhale, arch into a light backbend, and lift your face for kneeling cow; exhale and round your back, tucking chin to chest for kneeling cat. Repeat for several breaths. ● *Sweeter: Place a block between your heels to sit on, or slide a pillow or bolster between thighs and calves.*

Side stretch to the right, right hand on the mat, left arm reaching up and to the right. Stay several breaths. Switch sides. ● *Spicier: Bend the right elbow toward the ground as you side bend to the right.*

Open twist to the right, right hand on your hip or the mat, left hand on your outer right knee. Stay several breaths. Switch sides.

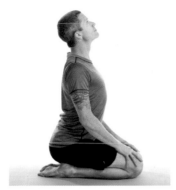

KNEELING COW

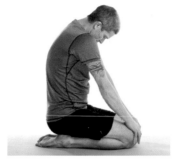

KNEELING CAT

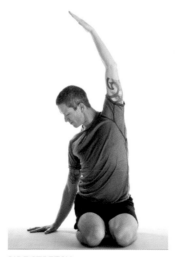

SIDE STRETCH

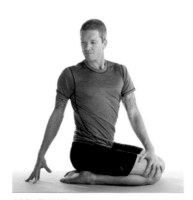

OPEN TWIST

SEATED WARM-UPS

# six moves of the spine, cross-legged

*Mobilize your shoulders and upper back.*

Sit cross-legged, then twist right for seated twist, resting your left hand on your right thigh. Stay several breaths.

Keeping your left hand on your right thigh, lift your right arm overhead, side bending to the left. Stay several breaths. Exhale and drop your right hand to your left knee, taking arms into an X in front of chest. Stay several breaths. Switch sides and return to seated twist.

Interlace your fingers overhead, palms upward. Relax your shoulders and lightly pull your hands away from each other while maintaining the clasp. Stay several breaths.

Exhale and round to a cat back, pushing your hands forward at shoulder height. Stay several breaths.

Interlace your fingers behind your back, resting your knuckles on the low back and squeezing elbows together. Lift your chest into a backbend for cow back. Stay for several breaths. ● *Spicier: In the backbend, lift your arms and straighten your elbows.*

Bend your elbows to move clasped hands to your right side waist, with the right elbow pointing back. Drop your right ear toward your right shoulder to feel a stretch in your left shoulder. Stay several breaths. Switch sides.

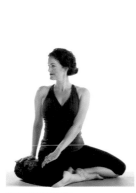

SEATED TWIST

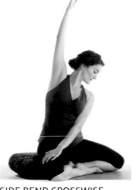

SIDE BEND CROSSWISE

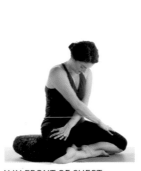

X IN FRONT OF CHEST

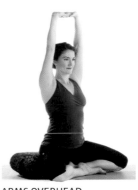

ARMS OVERHEAD

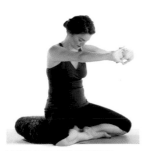

HANDS FORWARD WITH
CAT BACK

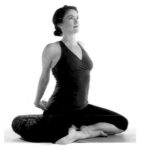

INTERLACED FINGERS BEHIND
BACK WITH COW BACK

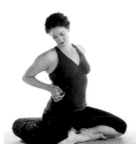

HANDS TO SIDE WAIST,
EAR TO SHOULDER

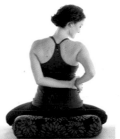

*alternate view*

PRONE

## six moves of the spine, prone

*Like a go-to weeknight recipe, this routine is quick, easy, and rewarding. It takes the spine in every direction and prepares for deeper movements.*

From child's pose, walk your hands to the right side until you feel a stretch. Stay several breaths. Switch sides.

Rise to your hands and knees. Inhaling, lift your tailbone, drop your belly, open your chest, and lift your gaze for cow. Exhaling, scoop your tailbone, round your back, pull your chin toward your chest, and drop the crown of your head toward the floor for cat. Repeat for several cycles.

On hands and knees, align your spine to neutral. Slide your right hand a few inches forward. Move your left hand to where your right hand was, dropping to your left elbow as you twist right to "thread the needle." Your right hand can come to your hip or lift upward for a chest stretch. Stay several breaths. Switch sides. ◉ *Sweeter: Stay on your left palm, elbow lifted, as you twist right.* ● *Spicier: Drop to your left shoulder.*

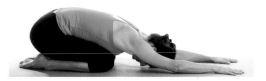

CHILD'S POSE

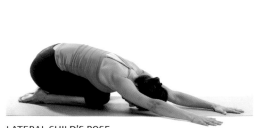

LATERAL CHILD'S POSE

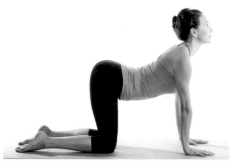

COW

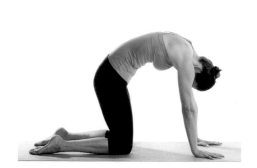

CAT

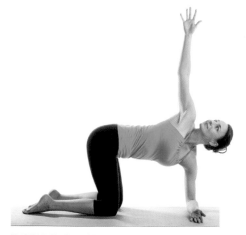

THREAD-THE-NEEDLE TWIST

# six moves of the spine, prone, leg extended

*The leg extension stretches the inner thigh and enables a different range of motion in the pelvis and spine.*

From table pose, extend your right leg to the right, in line with your hips and left knee, toes forward. Inhale to cow; exhale to cat. Repeat for several cycles.

Align your spine to neutral, drop your left elbow under your shoulder, and lift your right arm to your hip or to the ceiling as you twist to the right to "thread the needle." Stay several breaths. ● *Sweeter: Stay on your left palm as you twist right.* ● *Spicier: Drop to your left shoulder.*

Take both hands to the floor and walk your arms to the left until your left hand is in line with your left knee, fingers pointing away from the knee. Lift your right hand to your right hip, overhead, or over the left arm for reverse gate pose. Stay several breaths. ● *Seasoning: Draw big air-guitar circles around your body in both directions with your right arm.*

Repeat routine on the other side.

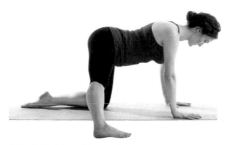

TABLE POSE, LEG EXTENDED

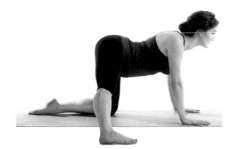

COW, LEG EXTENDED

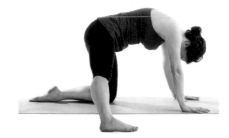

CAT, LEG EXTENDED

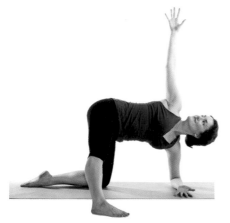

THREAD-THE-NEEDLE TWIST

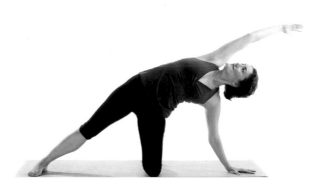

REVERSE GATE POSE

# six moves of the spine, prone, bent knee

*Stretches chest and hips while sharpening focus; try later in a practice as a cool-down.*

Lie on your belly and place your arms under your forehead, palms flat. Stay several breaths.

Slide your elbows under your shoulders, forearms parallel, for sphinx pose. Stay several breaths.

Bend your right knee for prone tree pose. Add a side bend by looking over your right shoulder toward your right knee. Stay several breaths. ● *Sweeter: Lower your chest back to the floor.* ● *Spicier: Straighten your left elbow to lift you deeper into the side bend.*

Square your shoulders forward, lift your right elbow, and slide your left arm to the right, palm up. Roll onto your outer left hip and leg and reach your right arm to the ceiling or to the floor behind you as you twist. ● *Sweeter: Keep your right hand on the ground.* ● *Spicier: Roll to your outer left hip, bend your left knee, and reach your right hand to left foot and/or straighten your right leg with right foot toward left hand.*

Return to center and switch sides.

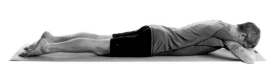

BELLY-DOWN CORPSE

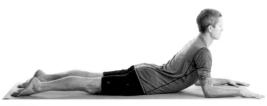

SPHINX

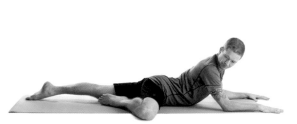

PRONE TREE POSE WITH SIDE BEND

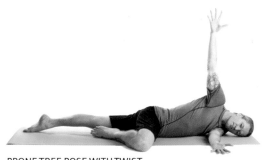

PRONE TREE POSE WITH TWIST

PRONE

# leg-swing flow

*The dynamic movements of this flow prep the body for the static holds. It's a good way to build heat and find release at the same time.*

Start in table pose. Keeping your right toes relaxed, inhale and roll over the toes to lift your right knee and press your right heel back, stretching toes. Exhaling, lower the right knee to the floor, returning to table pose. Repeat several rounds before holding the right knee off the ground for a calf stretch. ● *Sweeter: As you pulse, keep your toes curled and lower your right knee without touching the floor.*

From table pose, inhale and lift your right leg behind you as you arch your spine to cow back. Exhale and round to cat back, pulling your right knee toward your nose. Repeat several rounds.

Inhale and take your right leg straight behind you. Exhale and tap your right foot outside your left foot. Repeat several rounds before holding in the side bend. ● *Spicier: Lean your spine deeper to the left into the side bend.*

Return to table pose with the right leg extended behind you. Externally rotate from the hip so that your right knee and toes face to the right. Exhale and donkey kick your leg to the right; inhale and return to table pose with external rotation. Repeat several breaths, then lower your right foot to the floor in line with your left knee. Press into the left hand as you lift your right arm and twist toward the right. ● *Sweeter: Kick with a bent knee as you pulse.* ● *Spicier: Lower to your left elbow or shoulder as you twist.*

Return to center and switch sides.

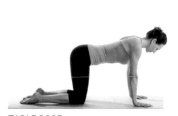

TABLE POSE

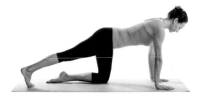

TOE STRETCH

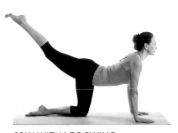

COW WITH LEG SWING

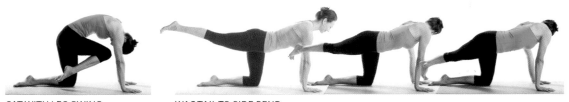

CAT WITH LEG SWING

WAG TAIL TO SIDE BEND

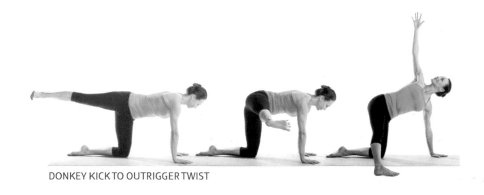

DONKEY KICK TO OUTRIGGER TWIST

SUPINE

## six moves of the spine, supine, one leg

*A lovely start to a mellow practice, this is also a great in-bed or post-workout routine.*

Start on your back, hugging both knees. Stay several breaths.

Slide your hands to your right knee and stretch your left leg toward the ceiling to stretch the hamstrings. Hold several breaths.

Keeping a firm hold on your right knee, slowly lower your extended left leg toward the floor, pausing with the heel a few inches from the mat to stretch the hip flexors. Stay several breaths. ◦ *Sweeter: Bend your left knee and rest your left foot on the floor.*

Guide your right thigh in slow circles in both directions.

Lower your right knee to the right in a reclining tree pose. Stay several breaths, then shimmy your shoulders to the right, arms reaching overhead, to stretch the left side for several more breaths. ◦ *Sweeter: Support the right thigh by sliding a blanket between thigh and floor.* ● *Spicier: Lightly tug on your left wrist or elbow as you side bend.*

Return your shoulders to align with your hips. Lift your bent right leg and cross your knee to the left as you roll onto the outer left hip. ● *Spicier: Straighten the bend in your right knee.*

Slowly circle your right arm around your body; move through several circles in one direction, then several more in the other. Finish with several breaths in stillness, reaching the right hand to the right.

Return to center and hug both knees. Repeat on the other side.

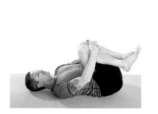
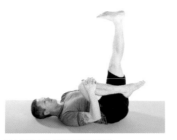
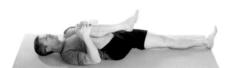

HUG KNEES

HAMSTRINGS STRETCH

HIP FLEXORS STRETCH

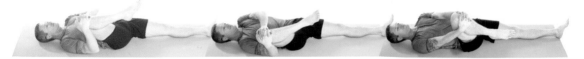

HIP CIRCLES

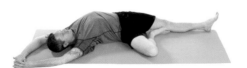

RECLINING TREE WITH SIDE BEND

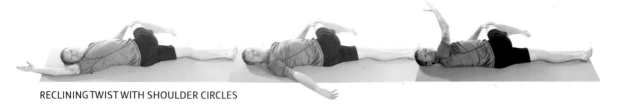

RECLINING TWIST WITH SHOULDER CIRCLES

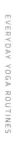

SUPINE

## six moves of the spine, supine, two legs

*Use this sequence to prepare for core work or as a stand-alone yoga snack.*

Start on your back, arms overhead in reclining mountain pose. Inhale and stretch your arms and legs away from each other; exhale and slacken your body. Repeat several rounds.

Cross your left ankle over your right ankle and shimmy your shoulders to the right to stretch the left side for banana. Hold several breaths. Switch sides.
● *Spicier: Tug on your left wrist or elbow with your right hand; swing your feet a few inches to the right.*

Hug your knees toward your chest. Stay several breaths.

Drop your feet to the floor, knees bent, hands by your hips. Inhale and lift your hips for bridge pose; exhale and lower. Repeat several rounds, then hold in bridge pose for several breaths. Finish by hugging your knees.

Slide your knees over your hips, hands to a T. Slowly lower your knees from side to side. Repeat several rounds, then lower both knees to the right, releasing them to the ground for a stretch; hold for several breaths. Switch sides. ● *Spicier: Straighten one or both knees as you lower and lift your legs.*

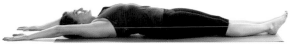

RECLINING MOUNTAIN

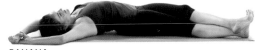

BANANA

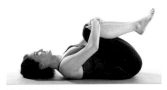

HUG KNEES

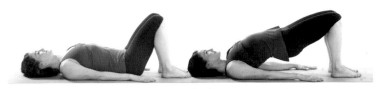

BRIDGE ARTICULATIONS
start

*finish*

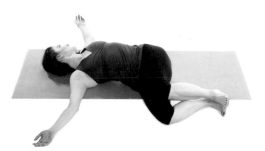

DOUBLE-KNEE TWIST

# standing routines for strength and balance |

Standing poses build whole-body strength, challenge your balance, and refine your awareness of where your body is in space. Think of them as the vegetables and lean protein of your practice: They do a lot of good for you.

FRONT OF THE MAT

## tall mountain flow

*A playful flow to refine your awareness of mountain pose and the ability to return to good form, this routine improves balance in space.*

Stand in mountain pose. Inhale and lift your arms overhead; exhale as you hug your belly to your spine and lower your shoulder blades down your back.

Inhale and lift your heels for tall mountain pose, balancing on the balls of your feet. Exhale and bend your knees as you lower your hips into a squat for chair pose.

Take another full breath as you lower your hips down to knee height, balancing on the balls of your feet for toe stand. Inhale and slowly rise all the way back to balance in tall mountain, heels high, arms overhead; exhale and return to mountain pose. ◉ *Sweeter: Omit the toe stand, squatting only as low as suits your knees and balance.* ◉ *Spicier: Extend one leg in front of you as you move through the cycle. To build strength, add several breaths at each stage of the cycle.*

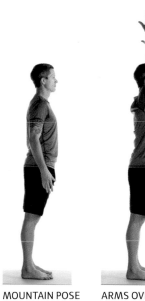
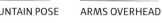

MOUNTAIN POSE

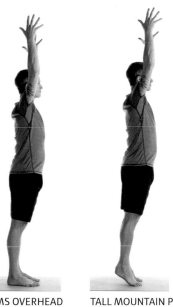

ARMS OVERHEAD

TALL MOUNTAIN POSE

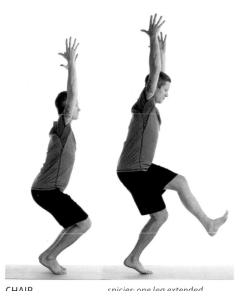

CHAIR

*spicier: one leg extended*

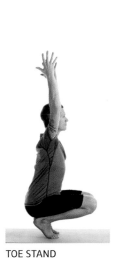

TOE STAND

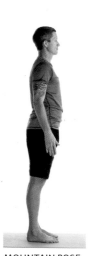

TALL MOUNTAIN POSE

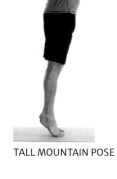

MOUNTAIN POSE

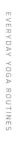

# parking lot yoga

*This sequence combines several standing poses without bringing the hands to the floor, meaning that it can be done mat-free in a parking lot (say, before a workout) as well as almost anywhere else.*

From mountain pose, inhale and lift your arms and right leg, knee to hip height for crane; exhale and step the right foot back for diagonal lunge, shoulders over left knee.

Inhale and lift your shoulders over your hips for crescent lunge; exhale and open to the right, dropping the right heel for warrior II.

Inhale and return to crescent lunge, lifting the right heel as you face forward; exhale and lean your torso to diagonal lunge. Inhale to pull through to crane; exhale and return to mountain pose. ● *Sweeter: Lift only the right heel, not the right thigh, to crane; slide the right foot along the mat as you step back to diagonal lunge. Lower your arms to prayer position to lighten the load on your shoulders. As you step forward, omit crane and simply move into mountain pose.* ● *Spicier: Depending on your needs, this sequence can be a dynamic warm-up (move on the half breath as outlined) or a strength-building practice (hold each pose for several breaths before moving to the next).*

Repeat the sequence on the other side.

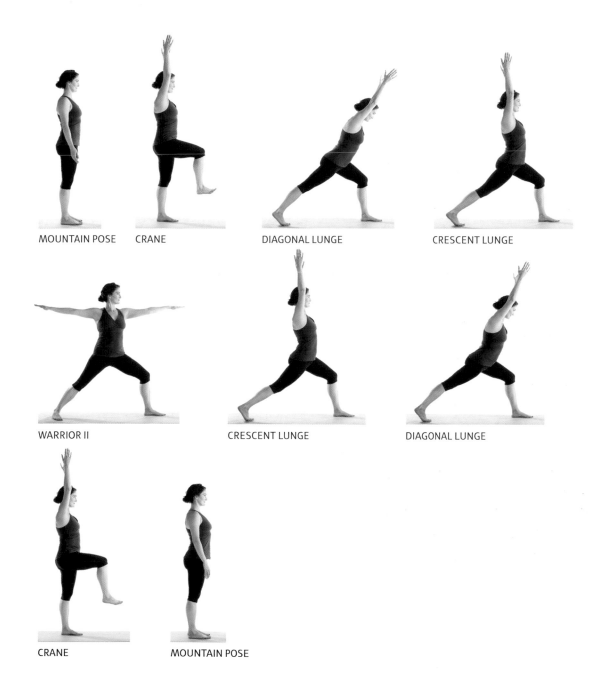

MOUNTAIN POSE    CRANE          DIAGONAL LUNGE          CRESCENT LUNGE

WARRIOR II                      CRESCENT LUNGE          DIAGONAL LUNGE

CRANE            MOUNTAIN POSE

FRONT OF THE MAT

# sun salutations

*A staple of most practices, sun salutations can be seasoned to your taste. Use them as a continuation of your warm-up or as the peak flow in your practice.*

Stand in mountain pose at the top of your mat. Inhale, raise your arms overhead; exhale, fold forward. Inhale, lift up halfway with your back long; exhale, reach your hands to the floor and step back to high plank. Inhale in high plank, then exhale for low plank. Inhale, upward-facing dog or cobra; exhale, downward-facing dog. Stay several breaths.

Inhale and step forward to halfway lift; exhale and forward fold. Inhale and rise to standing, arms overhead; exhale to mountain pose. Repeat several times. ⊙ *Sweeter: Keep your knees bent in the forward fold. Step one leg back to a lunge; hold for several breaths before moving to high plank. Drop your knees and move to knees-chest-chin, then cobra, or substitute with cat/cow. On the trip forward, use the same leg to step to a lunge on the other side, holding several breaths. ⊙ Spicier: On one exhalation, step or jump back through high plank to low plank, elbows close to your sides, torso hovering off the floor. Inhale and pull forward to upward-facing dog, hips off the mat; exhale and roll over your toes as you lift your hips to downward-facing dog.*

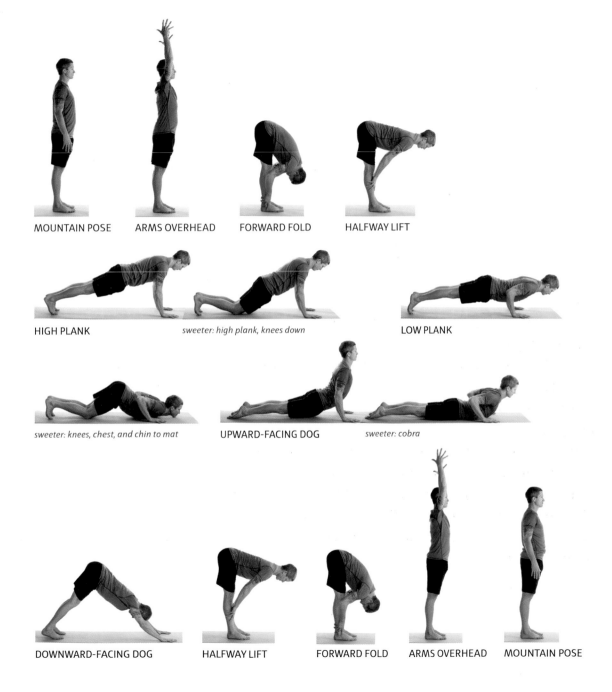

MOUNTAIN POSE     ARMS OVERHEAD     FORWARD FOLD     HALFWAY LIFT

HIGH PLANK     *sweeter: high plank, knees down*     LOW PLANK

*sweeter: knees, chest, and chin to mat*     UPWARD-FACING DOG     *sweeter: cobra*

DOWNWARD-FACING DOG     HALFWAY LIFT     FORWARD FOLD     ARMS OVERHEAD     MOUNTAIN POSE

# warrior I flow

*A mat-optional sequence that balances strength and flexibility in the legs and hips.*

Start in mountain pose at the back of your mat. Step your left foot forward and angle your right heel in slightly. Inhale to lift your arms; exhale to lunge your left knee just over your left ankle while keeping your right heel grounded. Hold for several breaths in warrior I.

Exhale and lean your torso over your left leg as you maintain the lunge. Hold for several breaths in diagonal warrior.

Inhale and bring your left knee toward straight, stopping when you feel the first edge of the hip and hamstring stretch. Hold several breaths in pyramid, your left knee straight but not locked. ● *Sweeter: Drape your spine over the left leg for a hamstring stretch.* ● *Spicier: Lift your torso and hold your spine parallel to the floor to build core and spine strength.*

Inhale and shift your weight into your left leg for warrior III; exhale and lean your chest forward as you lift your right leg behind you, arms reaching back or hands in prayer. Hold in warrior III for several breaths. ● *Sweeter: Keep your right toes on the floor, making a diagonal line from foot to head.* ● *Spicier: Lean your torso lower and lift your right leg toward parallel with the floor, hips square to the ground.*

Repeat the sequence on the other side. ● *Spicier: Pulse several times as you transition from pose to pose, then hold each pose for several breaths. The position of your arms in the last three poses will affect the intensity; for more challenge, reach your arms off your hips in an inverted V, off your shoulders in a T, or overhead in a V.*

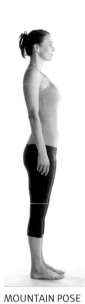

MOUNTAIN POSE

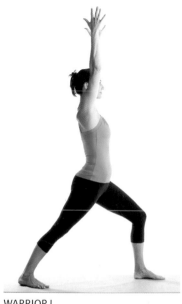

WARRIOR I

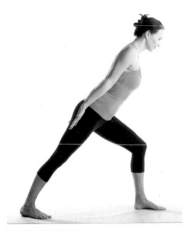

DIAGONAL WARRIOR

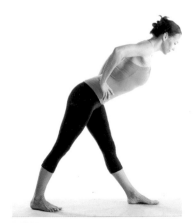

PYRAMID

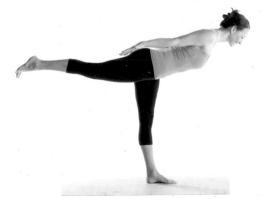

WARRIOR III

BACK OF THE MAT

# standing balance flow

*Use this five-pose routine to efficiently include the six moves of the spine and the four lines of the hip.*

Stand in mountain pose, shifting your weight to your left leg as you bend your right knee and hold your right foot with your right hand. Extend your left arm overhead and hinge from your hips as you kick your right foot behind you for dancer. Stay for several breaths.

Inhale and return to standing. Release your right foot and rest it against your left leg, anywhere other than against the knee. Spread your arms to your sides or lift them overhead, together or apart, for tree pose. Stay for several breaths.

● *Spicier: Add a side bend to the right, right palm or right elbow toward right thigh.*

Cross your right ankle over your left knee. Bend your left leg into a light squat, sending your hips back and down. Spread your arms for balance or, to stretch your chest, interlace your fingers behind your back and either squeeze your bent elbows together or straighten your arms. Stay in pigeon pose for several breaths.

Maintaining your squat with the left leg, cross the right knee tight over the left, inner thighs zipping together for eagle pose. Keep your arms spread or cross your left elbow over your right, resting the backs or the palms of the hands together. Stay for several breaths.

Repeat the sequence on the other side. ● *Sweeter: Take a break between poses, or do each pose first on the right leg, then on the left.* ● *Spicier: Eliminate breaks between poses; challenge your balance by slowly blinking your eyes or keeping them closed.*

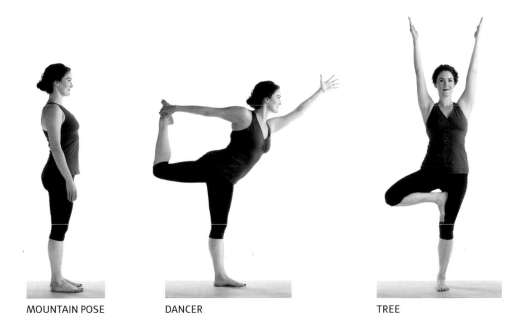

MOUNTAIN POSE          DANCER          TREE

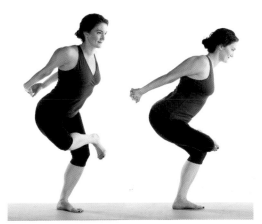

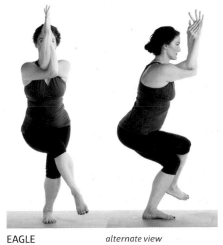

PIGEON          *alternate view*          EAGLE          *alternate view*

# warrior II flow

*This flow encourages balance between inner thigh and outer hip, which aids in knee health.*

Start in a wide stance. Inhale, lift your arms, and pivot your left toes left. Exhale, lower your arms parallel to the floor, and lunge your left knee just over the left ankle. Hold warrior II for several breaths.

Inhale, flip your left palm toward the ceiling, and lift your left arm as you lean back, resting your right hand lightly on your right hip or thigh. Stay in exalted warrior for several breaths.

Exhale and lean over your bent left leg, propping your left elbow on your left knee as you stretch your right arm over your left leg. Hold side angle for several breaths. ● *Spicier: Lower your left hand to a block or the floor, either just inside or just outside your left foot.*

Inhale, lift to center, and square your toes forward. Exhale and lean into a wide-angle fold, placing your hands on the floor beneath your shoulders. Stay in the fold for several breaths. Repeat on the other side. ● *Spicier: Pulse from pose to pose several times before holding a pose.*

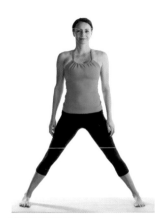

WIDE STANCE

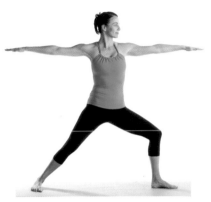

WARRIOR II

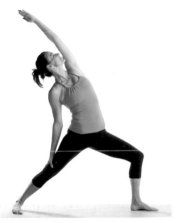

EXALTED WARRIOR

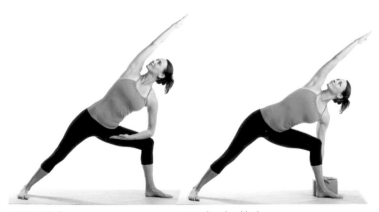

SIDE ANGLE

*spicier: hand on block*

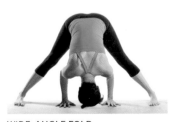

WIDE-ANGLE FOLD

# half moon flow

*An externally rotated variation on the warrior I routine, this builds strength and balance through the legs and core.*

From a wide stance, rotate your left foot left and lunge into your left knee for warrior II, arms reaching long. Hold the lunge for several breaths. ● *Seasoning: Pulse in and out of warrior II.*

Straighten your left leg and lean your torso over it, left hand to left leg and right hand reaching high, for triangle pose. Hold several breaths. ● *Seasoning: Pulse in and out of triangle pose.* ● *Spicier: Lean your torso without connecting your hand to your leg.*

Lean to stand on the left leg and lift the right leg for half moon pose, left hand to a block. Stay several breaths. ● *Seasoning: Pulse in and out before committing to half moon.* ● *Sweeter: Left hand to a block; right hand to hip.* ● *Spicier: Right hand to right foot, right knee bent.*

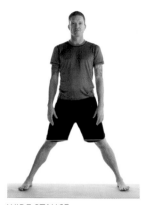

WIDE STANCE

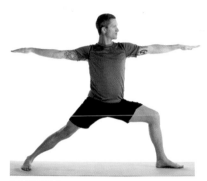

WARRIOR II

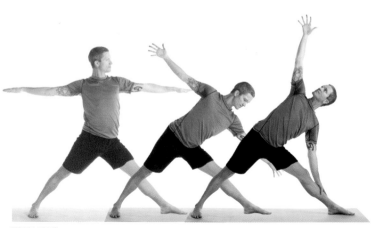

TRIANGLE

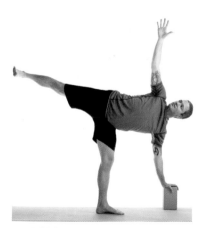

HALF MOON

# mat routines for core strength and hip flexibility |
Routines on the mat generally build core strength and hip flexibility. Think of them as the healthy carbohydrates in your practice: They nourish and ground you.

## side pigeon series

*Find deep release in the outer hips with this routine, which takes pigeon pose to new places.*

From downward-facing dog or table pose, inhale and lift your right leg behind you; exhale and round your back, pulling your knee toward your nose. Repeat several rounds of core plank swings, then step your right foot to your right pinky for lizard lunge. ◉ *Seasoning: Lower the back knee for more stretch; lift the back knee for more strength.*

Place your left palm under your left shoulder and walk your right leg in line with your hips as you rotate for side plank with a figure 4 leg. Stay several breaths.

Lower your left hip to the floor for side pigeon, taking several breaths to make the transition. Hold several breaths in the side bend.

Keeping your right foot down, spin to the right for a seated pretzel twist. Stay several breaths. ◉ *Sweeter: Step your right foot to the inside of your left leg.* ◉ *Spicier: Take the inner or outer left elbow across the right knee.*

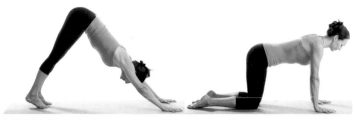

DOWNWARD-FACING DOG      *sweeter: table pose*

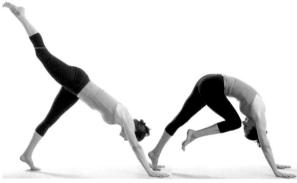 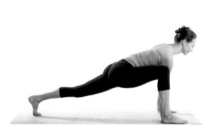

CORE PLANK SWINGS        LIZARD LUNGE

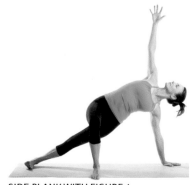 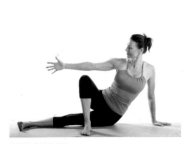 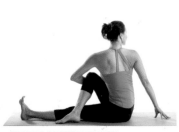

SIDE PLANK WITH FIGURE 4      SIDE PIGEON      SEATED PRETZEL TWIST

prone

# planks and backbends

*A go-to post-workout practice, this core-strengthening routine includes movement in every plane.*

Start in plank; hold several breaths. ● *Spicier: Repeat several rounds of alternating lifting one leg or one arm, moving with the breath.*

Lower to your belly and forearms. Bend your right knee, reach your right hand back to hold the top of your right foot, and kick into your hand as you lift for half bow. Hold several breaths. Rest on your belly before switching sides. ● *Sweeter: Keep your left elbow propped under your left shoulder for support.* ● *Spicier: Lift your left arm and leg for half locust on the left side and half bow on the right side.*

Bend both knees, reach both hands back to your feet, and then kick and lift to full bow; hold for several breaths. Rest in child's pose for several breaths.

Return to plank and pivot to the left hand, right hand reaching high, hips lifted for side plank. Hold for several breaths. ● *Seasoning: Drop your bottom elbow to the mat.* ● *Sweeter: Bend both knees, shins parallel to the back of the mat.* ● *Spicier: Stack your feet or lift your top leg.*

Drop to your left hip, loosely stack your knees, and spin to the left for an easy twist. Stay several breaths. Unwind and side bend to the right for mermaid. Switch sides and repeat from side plank.

Lift to reverse table pose for several breaths. ● *Sweeter: Keep your hips down but lift your chest.* ● *Spicier: Straighten your legs for reverse plank.*

From a seated position, finish by folding forward over your legs for several breaths.

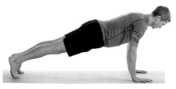
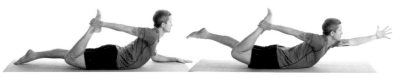

PLANK

HALF BOW

*spicier: half locust*

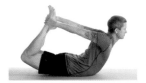
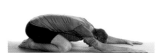

FULL BOW

CHILD'S POSE

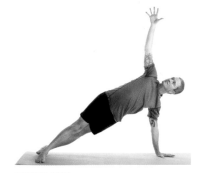
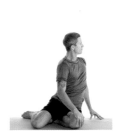
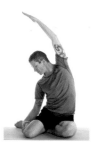

SIDE PLANK

EASY TWIST

MERMAID

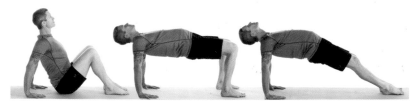
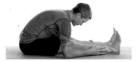

REVERSE TABLE POSE
start

*finish*

*spicier: reverse plank*

SEATED FORWARD FOLD

PRONE

# dancer/tree/pigeon/eagle

*This routine uses the standing balance flow as a model for core work on the mat— changing a pose's relationship to gravity changes its effect.*

Lie in sphinx pose, left forearm diagonal on the mat. Bend your right knee, reaching right hand to right ankle for half bow. ● *Sweeter: Pull your right heel toward your rear end for a quadriceps stretch with no kicking.*

Lift onto hands and knees. Step your right foot behind your left foot as you rotate into side plank on your left knee, right hand to the hip or the ceiling. Stay several breaths. Switch sides.

Lift onto hands and toes for a plank position. Push into your left hand and roll to the outer edge of the left foot for side plank as you step your right foot in front of your hips for a figure 4 shape. Reach your right arm high. Stay several breaths. Switch sides.

Come to your back. Cross left knee tight over the right, right elbow over the left. Inhale, lift your knees, shoulders, and head; exhale, pull your elbows and knees toward each other for eagle crunch. Complete several cycles of crunches before resting. Switch sides. ● *Sweeter: Keep your shoulders and head on the floor as you crunch, or support your head with your hands.*

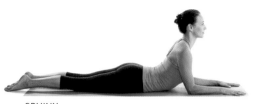

SPHINX

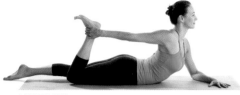

HALF BOW

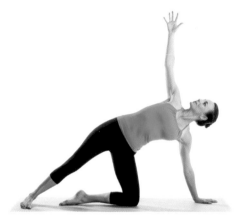

SIDE PLANK ON KNEE

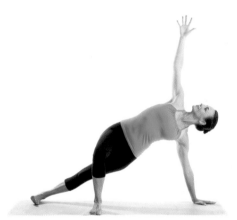

SIDE PLANK WITH FIGURE 4

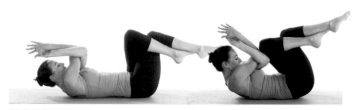

EAGLE CRUNCHES
*start*

*finish*

# table core

*This sequence strengthens the back and glutes while challenging your balance.*

Start on hands and knees in table pose. Extend your left arm and right leg for bird dog. ○ *Seasoning: Hold the extension for several breaths, or pulse: Inhale, extend your arm and leg; exhale, return to table pose.* Switch sides.

From bird dog, bend your right knee and catch your foot with your left hand. Stay in crossbow for several breaths. Switch sides.

Roll to side plank on the left knee, right foot behind left foot; stay several breaths. Lift your right leg for half moon on the knee; hold for several more breaths. Repeat on the other side. ○ *Sweeter: Move your right hand to the right hip and turn your gaze to the floor.* ● *Spicier: Reach your right hand high and turn your gaze to your right thumb.*

Finish with several breaths in child's pose.

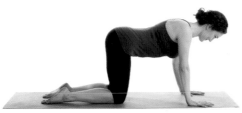

TABLE POSE

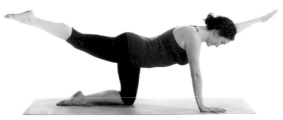

BIRD DOG

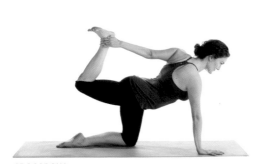

CROSSBOW

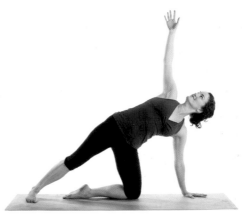

SIDE PLANK ON KNEE

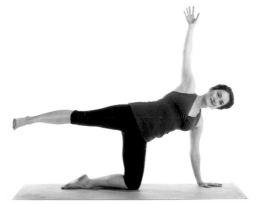

HALF MOON ON KNEE

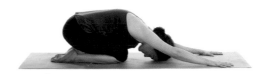

CHILD'S POSE

# core planks and lunges

*Build heat, cultivate upper-body strength, and release your hips in this*
*spicy routine.*

Start in downward-facing dog or table pose. Inhale and lift your left leg, keeping hips level. Exhale and shift to rounded plank, bringing your left knee toward your nose. Repeat several rounds of leg swings, then step your left foot between your hands for crescent lunge. Stay several breaths. Switch sides. ● *Sweeter: Leg swing from table pose. Keep your back knee down in crescent lunge, and place your hands to the floor or blocks.* ● *Spicier: Keep your back knee up and lift your hands to prayer or overhead to balance in crescent lunge. Between sides, flow from downward-facing dog to high plank to low plank to upward-facing dog and back to downward-facing dog.*

From downward-facing dog or table pose, inhale and lift your left leg; exhale and shift into plank, crossing your left knee toward your right elbow. Repeat several rounds, then extend your left foot to the right as you lift your right hand for side plank. Stay several breaths. Switch sides.

From downward-facing dog or table pose, inhale and lift your left leg. Exhale, shift to plank, and bring your left knee wide of your left elbow. Repeat several rounds, then step your left foot wide of your left hand for lizard lunge. Stay several breaths. Switch sides. ● *Seasoning: With your left knee and left toes pointing in the same direction, roll to the pinky-toe side of your left foot, rotating your torso to the left. Drop the right knee or lift it.*

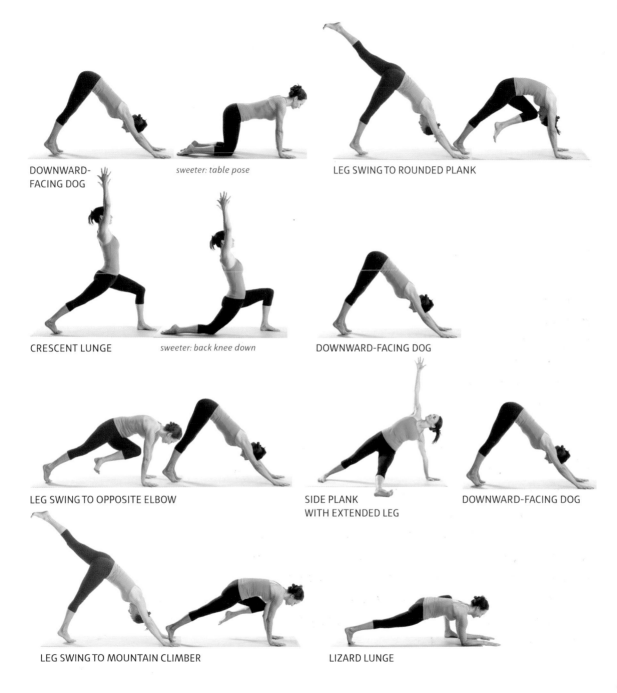

DOWNWARD-
FACING DOG

*sweeter: table pose*

LEG SWING TO ROUNDED PLANK

CRESCENT LUNGE

*sweeter: back knee down*

DOWNWARD-FACING DOG

LEG SWING TO OPPOSITE ELBOW

SIDE PLANK
WITH EXTENDED LEG

DOWNWARD-FACING DOG

LEG SWING TO MOUNTAIN CLIMBER

LIZARD LUNGE

# "Christina's World"

*This routine balances the musculature of the hips and calms the nervous system while releasing the muscles that support the spine. The prone twist position echoes the Andrew Wyeth painting.*

Start on hands and knees in table pose. Walk your left knee to meet your right knee, lowering your left hip to the ground. Twist and look over your left shoulder for prone twist. Stay several breaths. ● *Seasoning: Lower to your elbows or take your chest to the floor, arms spread wide.*

Lift your torso and move your right shin behind you, with the sole of the left foot near the right knee. Lean on a diagonal over your left leg onto your palms or elbows for a hip stretch. Stay in pinwheel pigeon for several breaths. ● *Seasoning: Lower your forehead to a block; angle your spine more to the left or more to the right.*

Keeping the pinwheel shape, lift your torso, push your left hand into the floor behind you, lift your hips, and point your toes as you arch into a backbend. Stay in wild camel several breaths.

Lower to the floor, and take several breaths in a wide-kneed child's pose. Repeat the sequence on the other side.

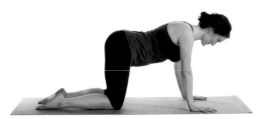

TABLE POSE

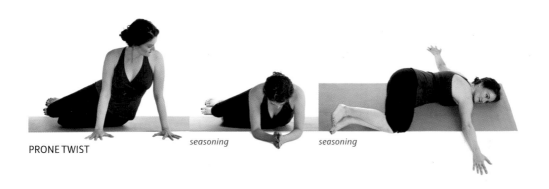

PRONE TWIST  *seasoning*  *seasoning*

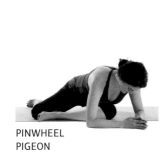

PINWHEEL
PIGEON

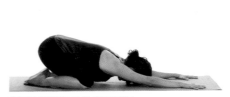

WILD CAMEL

WIDE-KNEED CHILD'S POSE

SEATED

# dynamic core

*Echoing moves from Pilates, this routine builds core strength and precision as it challenges all the abdominal muscles in both stabilization and articulation.*

Start sitting tall, legs extended. Exhale and slowly roll down to the floor. Inhale and lift your legs over your hips; exhale and roll your hips off the floor, legs overhead. Inhale to lower the hips to the floor; exhale and lower your legs to the mat. Inhale and roll up to seated staff; exhale and fold forward. Repeat several rounds. ● *Sweeter: Omit the rollover; keep your knees bent and hands to thighs throughout.* ● *Spicier: Lift your arms overhead as you roll up and down.* ● *Seasoning: Move slower. As you roll up and down and lift and lower your legs, pause in stages for a breath before moving a few more inches.*

Lying on your back, bring your legs over hips, spread your arms, ground your shoulders, and slowly tick-tock your knees from side to side. Repeat several rounds. ● *Sweeter: Keep your knees bent.* ● *Spicier: Straighten your legs; move slow and hold with your knees to the side.*

Lower your feet to the floor and lift your hips for bridge pose. Stay several breaths. ● *Sweeter: Press your hands to the floor.* ● *Spicier: Clasp your hands behind your back.*

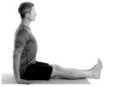

SEATED STAFF

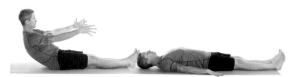

ROLL DOWN

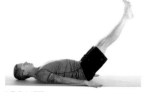

LEG LIFT

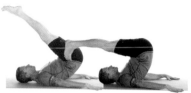

ROLL OVER

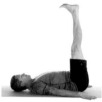

LOWER HIPS

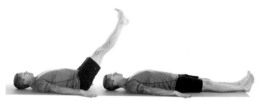

LOWER LEGS

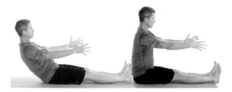

ROLL UP TO SEATED STAFF

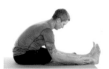

FORWARD FOLD

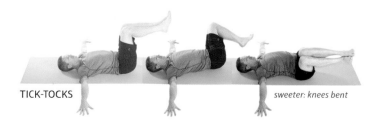

TICK-TOCKS

*sweeter: knees bent*

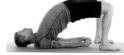

BRIDGE

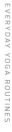

SEATED

# head-to-knee flow

*Release your hips and spine in every direction with this seated routine.*

Start seated, legs extended in front of you. Bend your right knee and set your right foot on the floor by your left knee. Turn to the right for pretzel twist, holding your right knee with your left hand or inner left elbow. Stay several breaths. ● *Spicier: Slide the outer left elbow to the outer edge of the right knee.*

Unwind from the twist and lower the right knee to the right, sole of the right foot against the left thigh. Fold forward over the left leg for head-to-knee pose; hold for several breaths.

Lift your torso and turn to the right, facing your bent right knee. Side bend over the left leg, reaching your right arm overhead. ● *Sweeter: Rest your right arm on your right hip or, reaching your forearm behind your back, on your left hip.* ● *Spicier: Lean more to the left, and stretch your right arm toward your left toes.*

Lift your torso and press your right hand into the floor. Lift your hips and point your right toes for side plank, resting on the right shin as you stretch the front of your left hip, left hand reaching over the left shoulder. ● *Sweeter: Rest your left hand on your left hip.* ● *Spicier: Reach your left hand over your right hand in a backbend.*

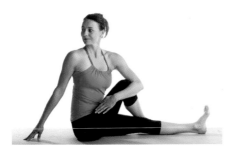

SEATED PRETZEL TWIST, LEG EXTENDED

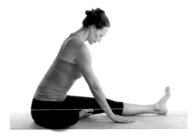

HEAD-TO-KNEE POSE

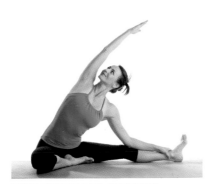

REVOLVED HEAD-TO-KNEE POSE

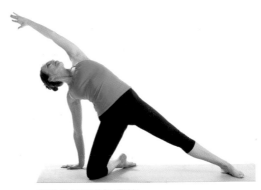

SIDE PLANK VARIATION

SEATED

# IT band flow

*Address the outer hips and iliotibial (IT) bands with this flow that spins you around your mat.*

Start sitting cross-legged, with your right foot by your left thigh. Spin right for seated pretzel twist, inner elbow to knee. Stay several breaths. ● *Sweeter: Hold your right knee with your left hand; straighten your left leg.* ● *Spicier: Take your outer left elbow to your knee.*

Unwind and lower your right knee over your left. Lift your left arm and bend your elbow; swing your right arm behind you and bend your elbow. Fold forward into cow-face fold for several breaths. ● *Seasoning: Use a strap to connect your hands behind your back, or reach your hands for each other.*

Release your hands to the left, lift to the balls of your feet, and pivot to lizard lunge, right knee outside your right hand. Stay several breaths. ● *Seasoning: Your left knee can be up or down; your torso can be higher or lower.*

Lift to the balls of your feet and make a quarter-turn left into a wide-legged forward fold. Plant your right hand under your face and spin left to twist. Hold several breaths; switch sides. ● *Seasoning: Lift your left hand to the sky; lunge your left knee.*

Reverse the sequence, walking left to lizard lunge, spinning forward for cow-face fold, and finishing in the seated twist.

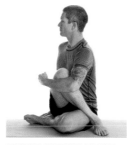

SEATED PRETZEL TWIST

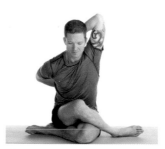

COW-FACE FOLD

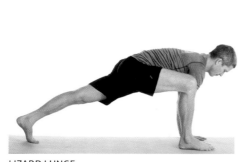

LIZARD LUNGE

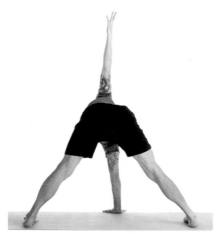

WIDE-LEGGED STANDING
FORWARD FOLD WITH TWIST

# folds and camel

*Move your spine in every direction as you release around the hips in this routine.*

Start with your legs in a wide straddle. Fold forward and stay for several breaths. ● *Sweeter: Prop your sitting bones on a blanket.*

Lean your torso over your right leg into a side bend. Stay several breaths. Switch sides. ● *Seasoning: Take your left hand to your left or right hip (reach behind your back).*

Lift to your knees. Move your right hand to your right hip as you stretch your left arm over your right shoulder and arch into a light backbend for a camel side stretch. Stay several breaths. Switch sides.

Take your hands to your lower back and lift your chest to camel pose. Stay several breaths. ● *Spicier: Lower your hands to your heels.*

Come to a wide-kneed child's pose. Slide your left arm under your right armpit to add a twist; rest on your forehead or left cheek. Stay several breaths. Switch sides.

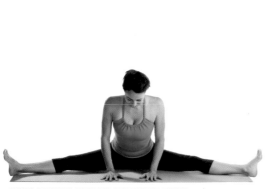

WIDE-LEGGED SEATED FORWARD FOLD

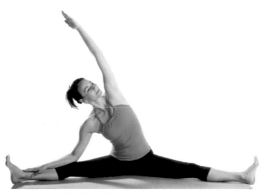

WIDE-LEGGED SEATED FORWARD FOLD WITH SIDE BEND

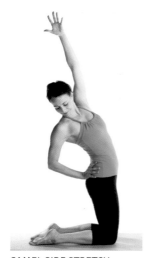

CAMEL SIDE STRETCH

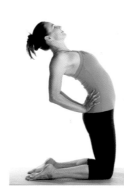

CAMEL

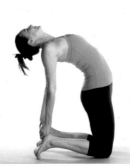

*spicier: hands to heels*

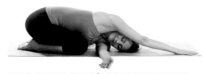

WIDE-KNEED CHILD'S POSE WITH TWIST

# table/boats/folds

*Builds core strength and hip flexibility after a workout and balances strength in the abs with strength in the back.*

Start seated, knees bent, hands behind you, fingers facing forward. Push into hands and feet and lift to reverse table pose. Stay several breaths. ● *Sweeter: Angle your hands differently if that suits your shoulders—fingers can face outward or even back.*

Lower your hips straight down. Lift your arms and legs to boat pose, keeping your chest open. Stay several breaths. ● *Sweeter: Keep your knees bent and hold the backs of your thighs.* ● *Spicier: Straighten your legs and lift your arms parallel to the floor, parallel to your legs, or overhead.*

Cross your ankles, lower your legs, and fold forward. Stay several breaths.

Return to reverse table pose for several breaths; release, then lift to boat pose, this time adding a twist. Inhale at center, exhale to twist to the side. Pulse several times.

Cross your ankles, opposite leg in front, and fold forward.

Lift up and return to reverse table pose. ● *Spicier: Return to reverse plank pose.* Stay for several breaths.

On your last trip to boat pose, alternate between boat and half boat: Inhale and lower your legs and torso toward the floor; exhale and lift back up to boat. Repeat several rounds.

Stretch your legs in front of you and fold forward for several breaths.

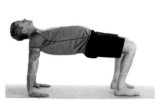 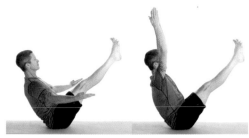

REVERSE TABLE POSE     BOAT POSE     *spicier: arms overhead*

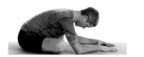 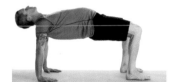 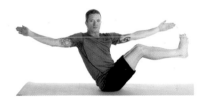

CROSS-LEGGED FORWARD FOLD     REVERSE TABLE POSE     BOAT WITH TWIST

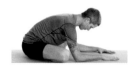 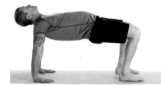 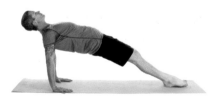

CROSS-LEGGED FORWARD FOLD     REVERSE TABLE POSE     *spicier: reverse plank pose*

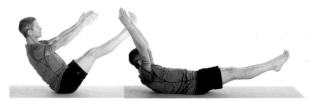 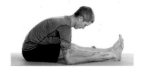

BOAT POSE     HALF BOAT POSE     STRAIGHT-LEGGED FORWARD FOLD

## strap stretches

*The floor supports your back while you stretch your legs, protecting your spine to focus release in your hips and thighs.*

Rest on your back with a strap around the ball of your left foot. Straighten your left leg until you find a hamstring stretch. Stay several breaths. ● *Sweeter: Bend your right knee and rest your right foot on the ground.*

Bend your left knee toward your left armpit for half happy baby. Push your right heel away from center to release the front of the right hip. Stay several breaths.

Move the strap to your left hand and, keeping your right leg active, straighten your left knee as you drop your left leg to the left. Stay several breaths.

Returning to center, keep your left hip on the ground as you move the strap to your right hand and cross your left leg to the right for an iliotibial (IT) band and outer hip stretch. Stay several breaths.

With the strap still in your right hand, roll to the outer right hip as you cross your left leg over and twist your spine. ● *Sweeter: Bend your left knee, holding the outer knee with your right hand.* ● *Spicier: Keep your left shoulder on the floor and turn your gaze left.*

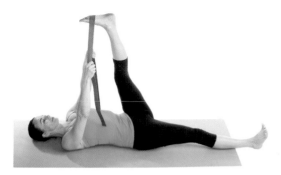

HAMSTRING STRETCH

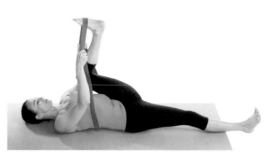

HALF HAPPY BABY

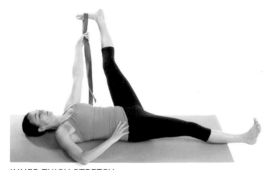

INNER-THIGH STRETCH

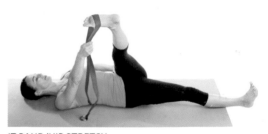

IT BAND/HIP STRETCH

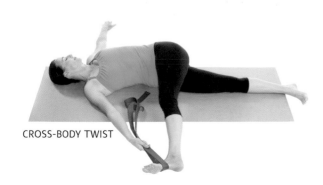

CROSS-BODY TWIST

SUPINE

# reclining twists

*Balances the musculature around your hips and releases the spine.*

Lie on your back, knees bent. Cross your right ankle over your left knee for figure 4. Stay several breaths. ◉ *Seasoning: Pull your legs toward your chest; drop your knees an inch or two to either side.*

Pull your left heel to your right hip as you lower the figure 4 to the left. Rest your right foot on the floor or your left thigh for supine pretzel twist. Stay several breaths. ◉ *Spicier: Reach your hands toward opposite ankles.*

Move the entire figure 4 unit to the other side, pointing your knees right as you rest on the inner edge of the left foot for reverse supine pretzel twist. Stay several breaths. ◉ *Sweeter: Drop your right foot to the floor and pull your left knee closer to your right knee.* ◉ *Seasoning: Lift one or both arms along the floor overhead.*

Cinch your knees together, right knee tight over left, and drop your knees to the left for a cross-legged twist. Stay several breaths. ◉ *Sweeter: Uncross the legs or bolster them from below.* ◉ *Spicier: Keep your right shoulder down as you turn your gaze to the right.*

Switch sides and start from the beginning.

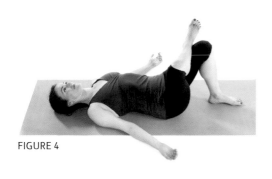

FIGURE 4

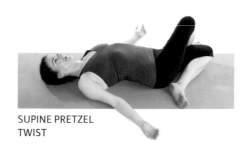

SUPINE PRETZEL
TWIST

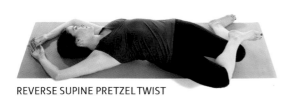

REVERSE SUPINE PRETZEL TWIST

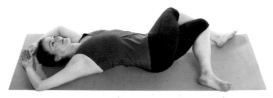

CROSS-LEGGED TWIST

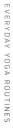

# wall series

*Enjoy the benefit of inversion and release of your hips in this multitasking routine.*

Start with your legs up the wall. Pull your left leg toward your torso, rolling your ankle a few times in each direction. Lightly hold your left thigh with your hands as you stay several breaths in the hamstring stretch.

Bend your left knee and drop it to the left armpit for half happy baby. Stay several breaths. ● *Sweeter: Rest your left foot on the wall.*

Keeping your left knee bent, cross your outer left ankle over your right thigh for figure 4. Stay several breaths. ● *Spicier: Flip the sole of your right foot to the wall and bend your right knee.*

Repeat on the other side.

If your upper back and neck are healthy, bend both knees and lift your hips for bridge pose at the wall. Your hands can support your lower back. Stay several breaths before lowering slowly.

Drop both knees to the right, feet to the base of the wall. Stay several breaths in the twist, then repeat on the other side. ● *Sweeter: Scoot a few inches away from the wall.*

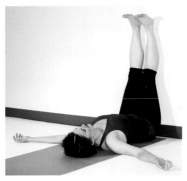

LEGS UP THE WALL

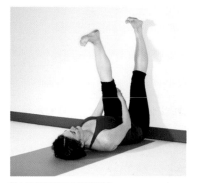

HAMSTRING STRETCH

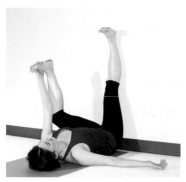

HALF HAPPY BABY

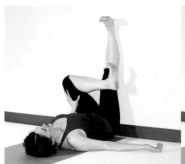

FIGURE 4

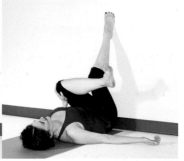

*spicier: right knee bent*

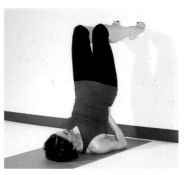

BRIDGE/HALF SHOULDERSTAND

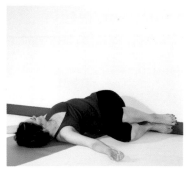

DOUBLE-KNEE TWIST

HIP RESET

## bridge to block

*Especially useful when you've spent much of the day sitting, this routine targets your hip flexors.*

Slide a yoga block or stack of pillows under your pelvis for a supported bridge pose. Make sure the support is under the bony back part of your pelvis and tops of your glutes. Stay several breaths to settle.

As you grow comfortable, stretch your legs and arms away from each other. Stay several more breaths.

With your right hand, hug your right knee toward your chest as you press out through your left leg and reach your left arm along the floor overhead. Stay several breaths. Switch sides.

Bend your knees and push your feet into the floor to lift your hips; remove the block, lower your hips, and hug your knees toward your chest.

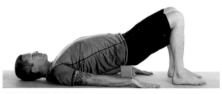

BRIDGE TO BLOCK

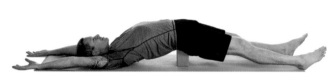

STRETCH LONG ON BLOCK

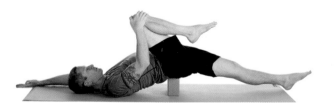

HUG KNEE ON BLOCK

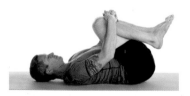

HUG KNEES

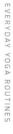

HIP RESET

# cow-face/cobbler

*Balance the inner and outer lines of your legs in this two-pose hip reset.*

Lie on your back. Cross your left knee tight over your right knee and hug both knees toward your chest for reclining cow-face. Stay several breaths. Switch sides. ● *Sweeter: Cross at the ankles instead of the knees.* ● *Spicier: Slide your hands toward opposite ankles, swiveling ankles toward opposite hips.*

Slide the soles of your feet together as your knees lower toward the floor for reclining cobbler. Spread your arms to an inverted V, a T, or a diamond shape overhead. ● *Sweeter: Support your knees from underneath with blocks or pillows. Use a pillow for your head.*

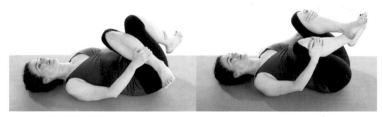

RECLINING COW-FACE

*sweeter: cross ankles*

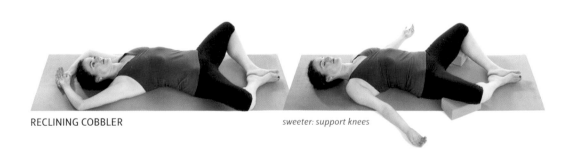

RECLINING COBBLER

*sweeter: support knees*

SPINE RESET

# backbends and happy baby

*Choose the degree of backbending that suits your energy.*

Rest on your back with your knees bent, hands by your hips. Push into your feet and lift your hips for bridge pose. Stay several breaths. ◦ *Sweeter: Slide a block under your pelvis for supported bridge.* ◦ *Seasoning: Tuck your shoulder blades toward your spine; interlace your fingers behind your back, pushing pinkies into the mat.*

Take your hands to the floor, fingers pointed to your shoulders, elbows bent over wrists. Lift the lower part of your body to bridge, then press into your hands, straighten your arms, and lift your upper body for upward-facing bow. Stay several breaths. ● *Spicier: Lift one leg, knee bent or leg straight. Switch sides.*

Bring your knees toward your armpits for happy baby. Stay several breaths. ◦ *Seasoning: Hold the backs of your knees, your ankles, or your feet; rock side to side.*

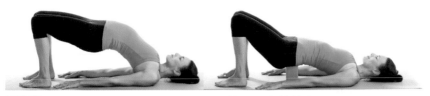

BRIDGE                           *sweeter: supported bridge*

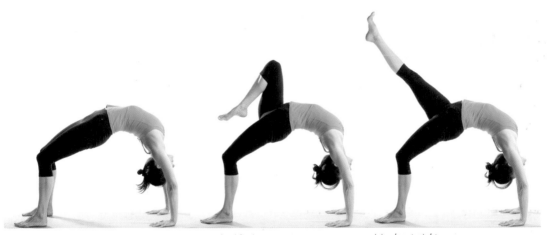

UPWARD-FACING BOW          *spicier: leg lifted*          *spicier: leg straight*

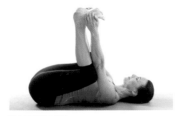

HAPPY BABY

SPINE RESET

# unsupported inversions

*Builds stamina and new levels of concentration and focus.*

From your back, lift your hips and roll your weight to your shoulders—not your neck and head—as you lift to shoulderstand for several breaths. ◉ *Seasoning: Slide a blanket under your shoulders; bend your knees.*

Bend your knees and lower your feet behind your head for plow. Stay several breaths. ◉ *Sweeter: Keep your hands on your low back.* ◉ *Spicier: Clasp your hands on the floor, or reach your hands toward your feet.*

Roll your hips back to the mat, extend your legs, and push into your forearms as you puff your chest for fish pose. Stay several breaths. ◉ *Sweeter: Bend your knees.* ◉ *Spicier: Lift your legs and arms as though for boat pose.*

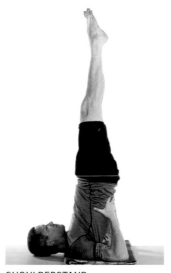

SHOULDERSTAND

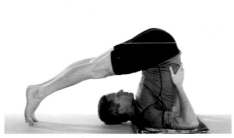

PLOW
*sweeter*

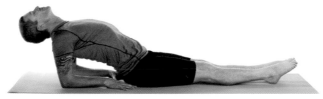

FISH

SPINE RESET

# supported inversions

*A gentler approach to inversions uses props to achieve a calming effect and spinal reset.*

Start in bridge pose on the block. Lift your legs over your hips for supported shoulderstand. Stay several breaths.

Bend your knees and drop them toward your shoulders. Stay in bent-knee plow for several breaths. ● *Spicier: Roll your hips off the block.*

Slide the block under your back with its top edge along the lower tips of your shoulder blades in supported fish. Stay several breaths. ● *Seasoning: Spread your arms.* ● *Sweeter: Add a pillow for your head.*

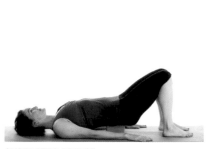

SUPPORTED BRIDGE

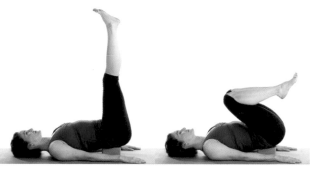

SUPPORTED SHOULDERSTAND  *sweeter: legs bent*

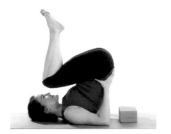

BENT-KNEE PLOW
*spicier*

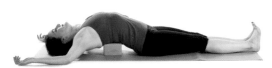

SUPPORTED FISH
*seasoning*

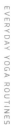

NERVOUS SYSTEM RESET

# legs up the wall

*The inversion of your legs helps reduce swelling and calms your nervous system.*

Sidle close to the wall and prop your heels against it for legs up the wall. Or add a block under the pelvis for supported legs up the wall. ● *Sweeter: Use a bolster to support your pelvis.*

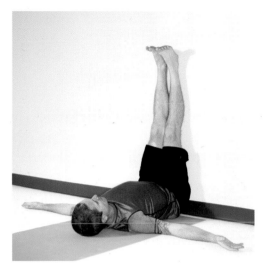

LEGS UP THE WALL

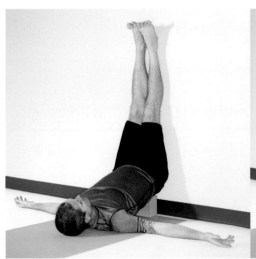

SUPPORTED LEGS UP THE WALL

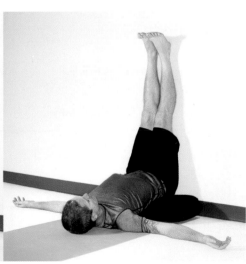

*sweeter: with bolster*

NERVOUS SYSTEM RESET

# restorative six moves of the spine

*Luxuriate in these poses for several minutes each. Use props to fill in any space between you and the floor; add an eye bag in supported cobbler if you have one.*

Recline on a bolster or a pile of pillows, hips on the ground, knees wide, and feet together. ● *Sweeter: Prop your knees from below.*

Twist with your belly to the bolster, knees bent. Switch sides.

Turn the bolster and side bend over it, adding cushioning for your head as needed. Switch sides.

Take your knees wide on either side of the bolster as you rest your belly and chest on it for child's pose.

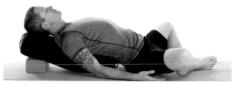

SUPPORTED COBBLER

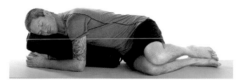

TWIST TO BOLSTER

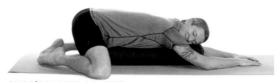

SIDE BEND TO BOLSTER

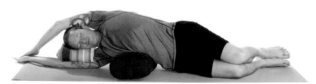

CHILD'S POSE TO BOLSTER

NERVOUS SYSTEM RESET

## corpse pose

*Even if you're here for only one minute, be sure to enjoy this close to your practice; it's the truffle after a satisfying meal.*

Stretch long on your mat, arranging your legs, pelvis, spine, and arms so you can feel completely relaxed. Stay several minutes. ● *Sweeter: Add props to fill the space between the body and the floor, especially at the backs of the knees and as a pillow. Add a blanket for warmth and weight. Add an eye pillow for darkness.*

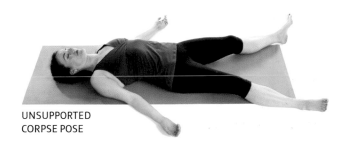

UNSUPPORTED
CORPSE POSE

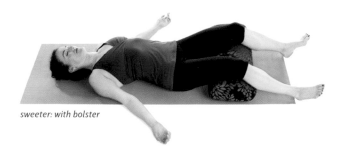

*sweeter: with bolster*

BREATH AWARENESS AND MEDITATION

# breath in space

*Try this breath exercise in one of the positions pictured to experience different relationships to gravity. Include it before, during, and after your practice.*

Get comfortable and tune in to how your breath is moving in the space of your body. Notice where it enters and what its temperature is at both entry and exit. Notice the farthermost point at which you feel the breath. Notice what moves as your inhalation continues, how it feels to be full of breath, what moves as your exhalation continues, and how it feels to be empty of breath. Continue this awareness for several minutes.

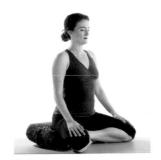

SEATED

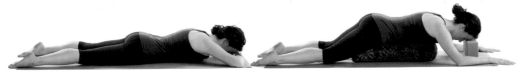

BELLY-DOWN CORPSE

*sweeter: with bolster and block*

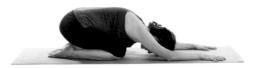

CHILD'S POSE

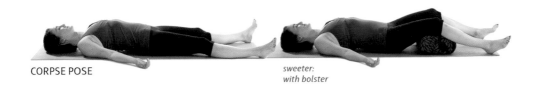

CORPSE POSE

*sweeter:
with bolster*

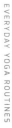

BREATH AWARENESS AND MEDITATION

# breath in time

*When you watch how your breath moves across time, it usually deepens and lengthens in response.*

Get comfortable and tune in to how long it takes for you to breathe. Notice the length of your inhalations and the length of your exhalations. Notice the length of the pause between inhalation and exhalation and the length of the pause between exhalation and inhalation. Continue for several minutes.

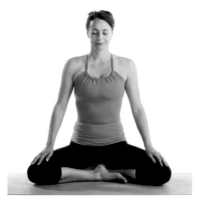

SEATED

# counting meditation

*Don't be alarmed if you find it tough to maintain focus even to count to 10.*
*Your ability to sustain attention in the moment will grow with practice.*

Get comfortable and choose a number from 10 to 50 to count toward. Inhaling,
think one; exhaling, think one. Inhaling, think two; exhaling, think two. Continue
until you reach the number or until you lose focus, at which point you can start
again from one. Continue for several minutes—use a timer to keep you honest.
● *Seasoning: Count each half of the breath, inhaling "one," exhaling "two."*
*Or count from a bigger number back down to one.*

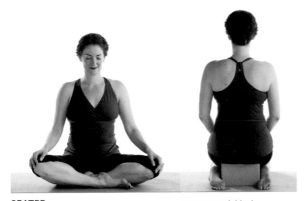

SEATED                    *sweeter: with block*

BREATH AWARENESS AND MEDITATION

# mantra meditation

*A mantra is a tool to focus the mind. It can be a personally meaningful phrase, a prayer, or a word, like "peace."*

Get comfortable and choose a mantra—a word, phrase, or verse to repeat to yourself. Repeat the mantra silently or out loud, developing a rhythm that helps focus your mind. Continue for several minutes—use a timer to keep you honest.
● *Seasoning: Coordinate the mantra with your breath.*

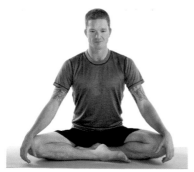

SEATED

# three-part breath

*Gain finesse in your breathing by isolating the movements of inhalation and exhalation into three parts. Feel the movement that accompanies your breath in the belly, ribcage, and upper chest as the three regions.*

Get comfortable and bring your attention to your breath. Bring in your inhalation a third of the way, then pause briefly. Continue to inhale to two-thirds full, then pause. Finish by inhaling completely, then pause. Exhale in three parts, as well. Continue for several rounds and release. ◉ *Sweeter: Divide the inhalation into three parts, but keep the exhalation continuous and smooth, or enjoy a continuous inhalation and pause over the course of a three-part exhalation.* ◉ *Seasoning: Feel the breath enter from the top down, noticing the movement of inhalation in the upper chest, ribcage, then belly, and the reverse on exhalation. Or take the reverse, feeling inhalation moving upward, first in the belly.*

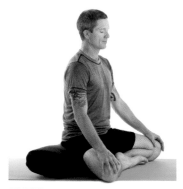

SEATED

restorative cool-downs

# extended exhalation

*This exercise helps engage the parasympathetic nervous system's relaxation response, making it ideal for calming yourself or unwinding before bed.*

Observe a few rounds of breath, comparing the length of the inhalation with the length of the exhalation. Count the beats of the inhalation, and extend the exhalation to last several beats longer (e.g., follow an inhalation of a count of 6 with an exhalation of a count of 8 or 10). Continue for several rounds and release.

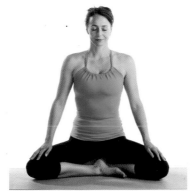

SEATED

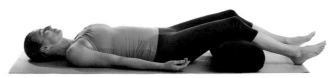

SUPINE

# everyday yoga
# practices

Here are ways to combine the routines from Part 2 into complete practices. The short practices will take 10 to 20 minutes to complete; the long ones will take 50 to 80 minutes. Each practice targets a different area—core, lower body, and so on. Round out each practice by including one or more breath exercises or meditations.

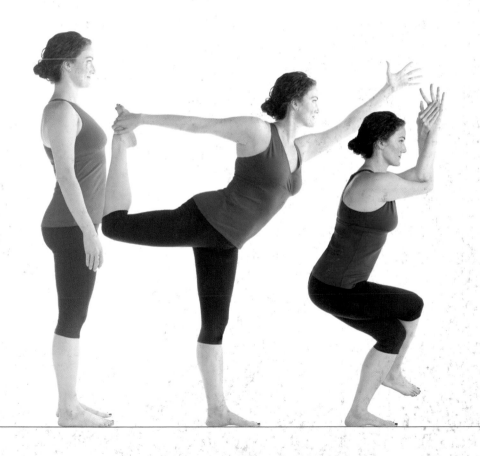

# core strength and stability

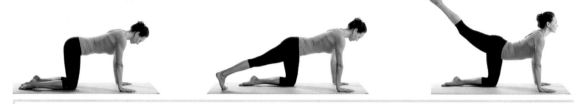

leg-swing flow  p. 36

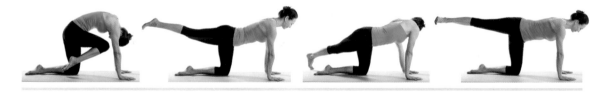

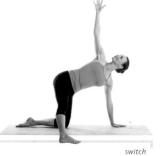

*switch sides*

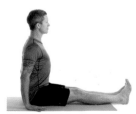

dynamic core  p. 68

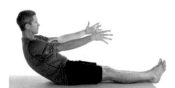

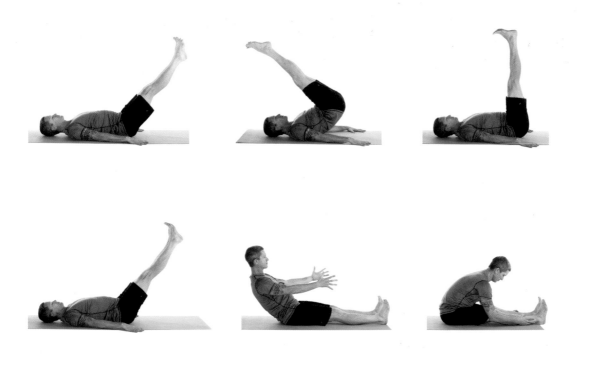

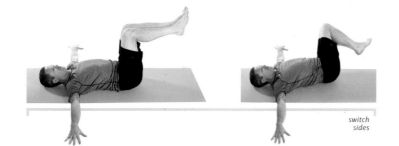

*switch sides*

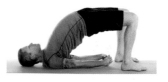

# lower-body strength and stability

short practices

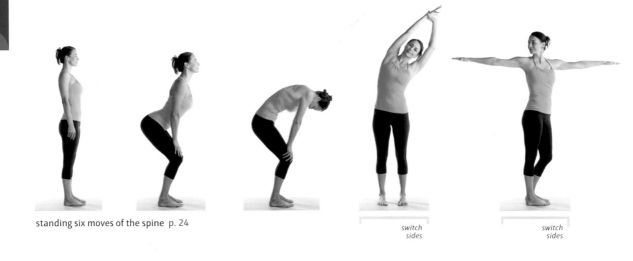

standing six moves of the spine  p. 24

*switch sides*

*switch sides*

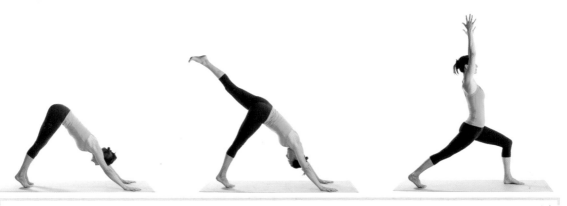

core planks and lunges  p. 64

*switch sides*

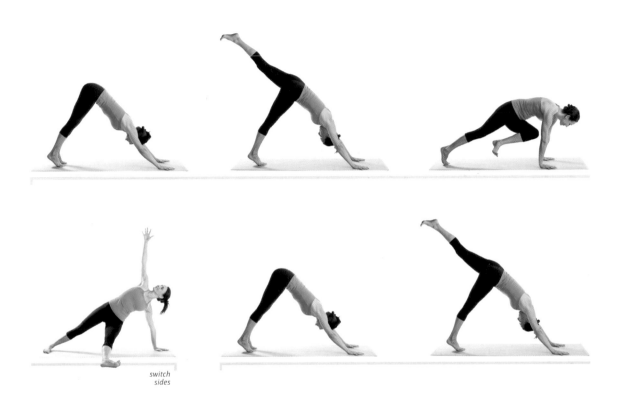

*switch
sides*

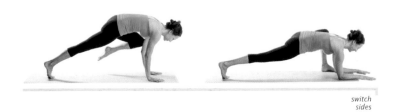

*switch
sides*

# lower-body flexibility and mobility

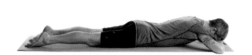

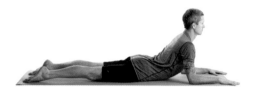

six moves of the spine, prone, bent knee  p. 34

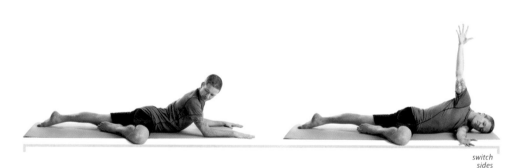

*switch
sides*

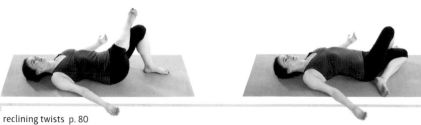

reclining twists  p. 80

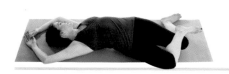 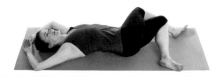

*switch sides*

# upper-body strength and stability

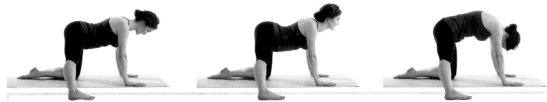

six moves of the spine, prone, leg extended  p. 32

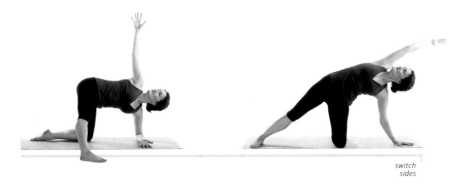

switch
sides

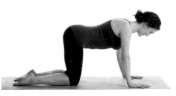

table core  p. 62

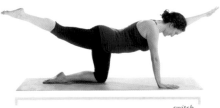

switch
sides

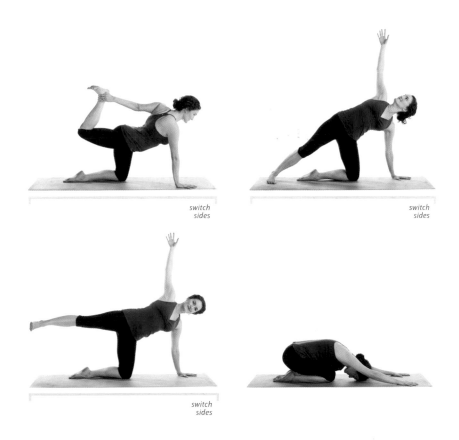

*switch sides*

*switch sides*

*switch sides*

# upper-body flexibility and mobility

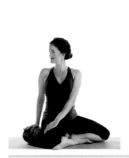 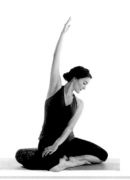 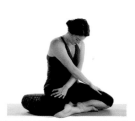

six moves of the spine, cross-legged  p. 28

*switch
sides*

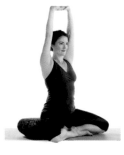 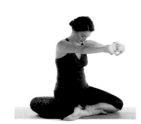 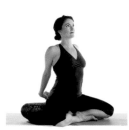

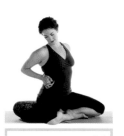 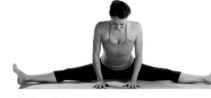 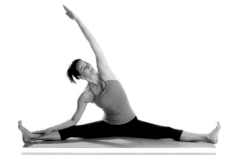

*switch
sides*

folds and camel  p. 74

*switch
sides*

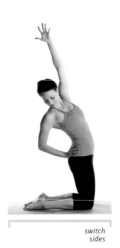

*switch
sides*

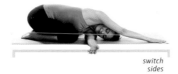

*switch
sides*

# relaxation and recovery

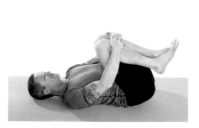
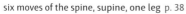
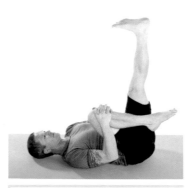

six moves of the spine, supine, one leg  p. 38

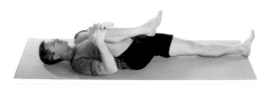
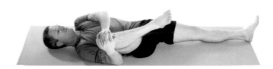

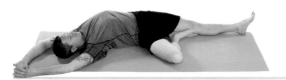
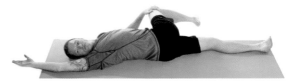

*switch sides*

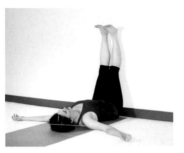 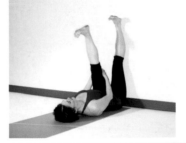 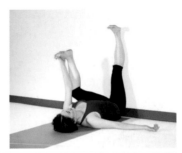

wall series  p. 82

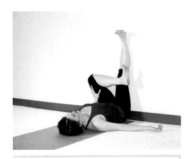 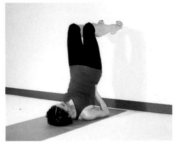 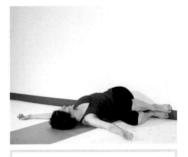

*switch sides*

*switch sides*

## whole-body balance

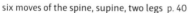

six moves of the spine, supine, two legs  p. 40

*switch sides*

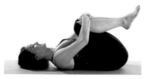
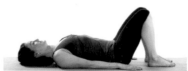
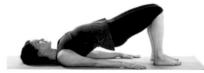

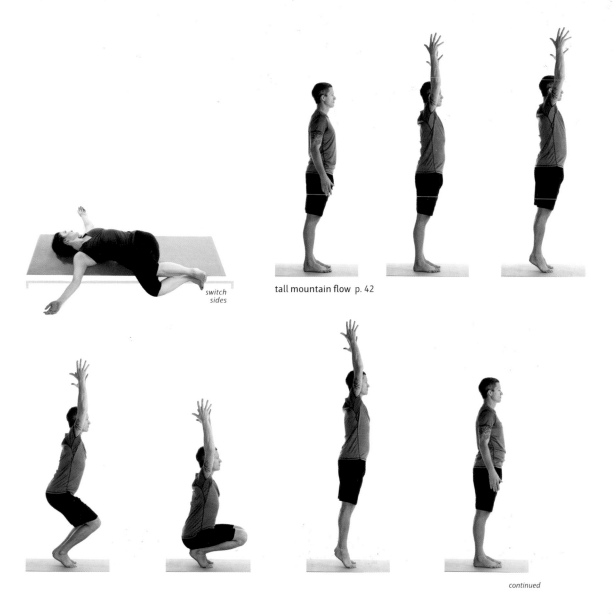

*switch
sides*

tall mountain flow  p. 42

*continued*

123

# whole-body balance *continued*

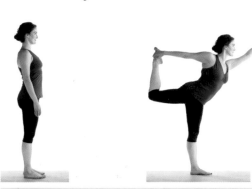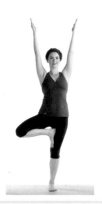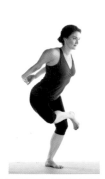

standing balance flow  p. 50

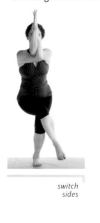

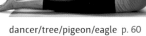
*switch sides*

dancer/tree/pigeon/eagle  p. 60

*switch sides*

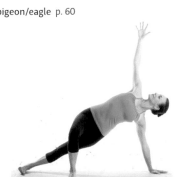
*switch sides*

*switch sides*

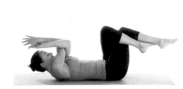
*switch sides*

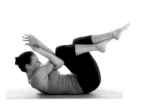
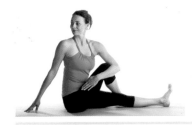
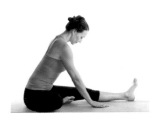

head-to-knee flow p. 70

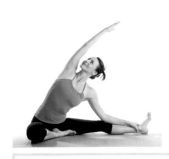
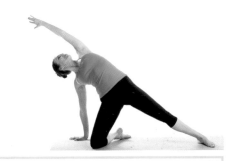

switch
sides

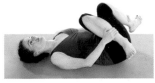
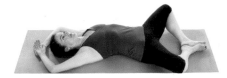

cow-face/cobbler p. 86    switch
sides

# core strength and stability

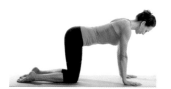
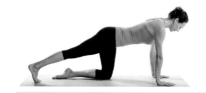
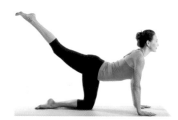

leg-swing flow  p. 36

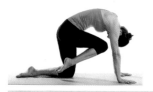
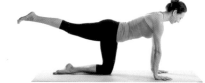
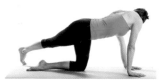

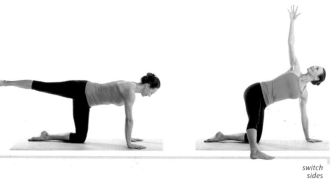
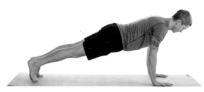

*switch
sides*

planks and backbends  p. 58

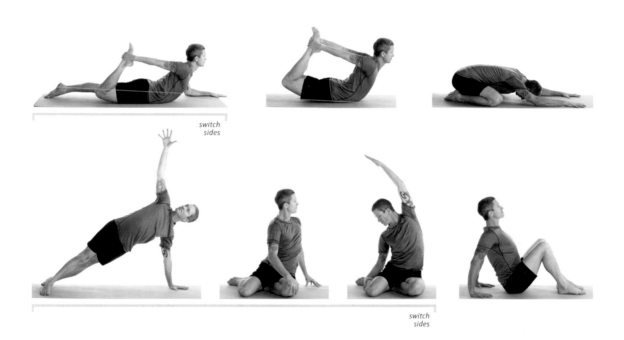

*switch
sides*

*switch
sides*

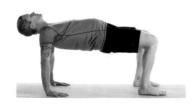

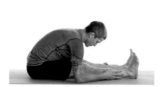

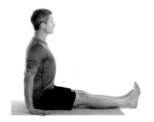

dynamic core  p. 68     *continued*

# core strength and stability *continued*

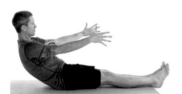
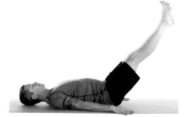
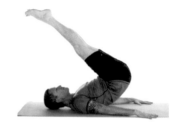

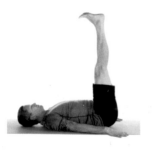
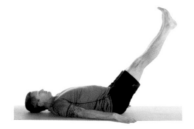
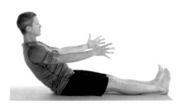

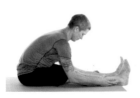
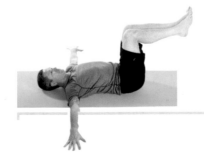
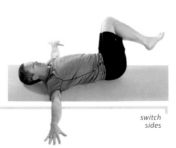

*switch
sides*

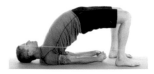 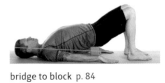 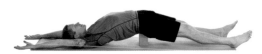

bridge to block  p. 84

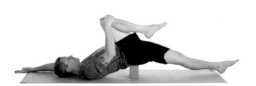  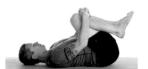 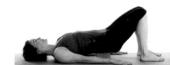

*switch sides*

supported inversions  p. 92

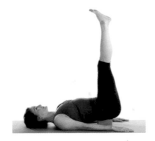 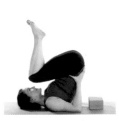 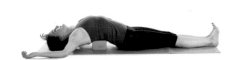

# lower-body strength and stability

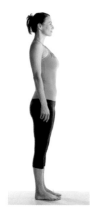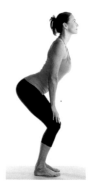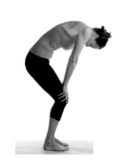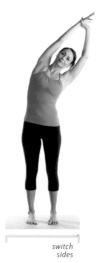

standing six moves of the spine  p. 24

*switch sides*

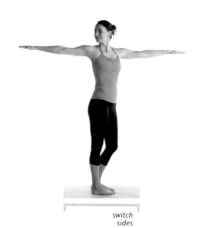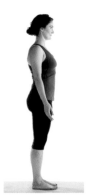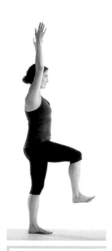

*switch sides*

parking lot yoga  p. 44

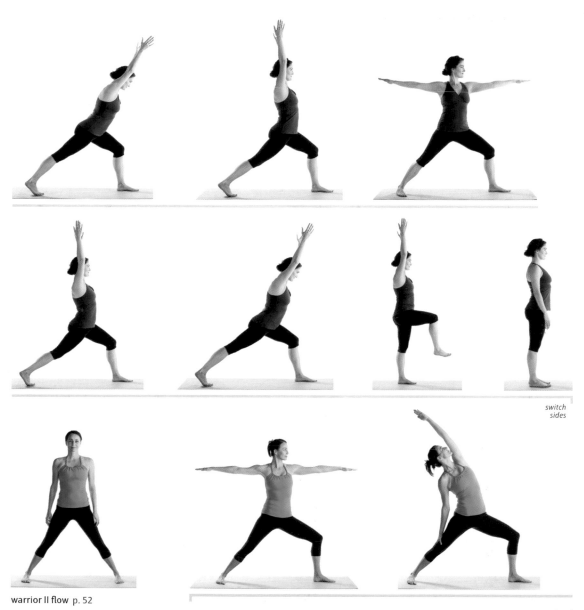

*switch
sides*

warrior II flow  p. 52

*continued*

# lower-body strength and stability *continued*

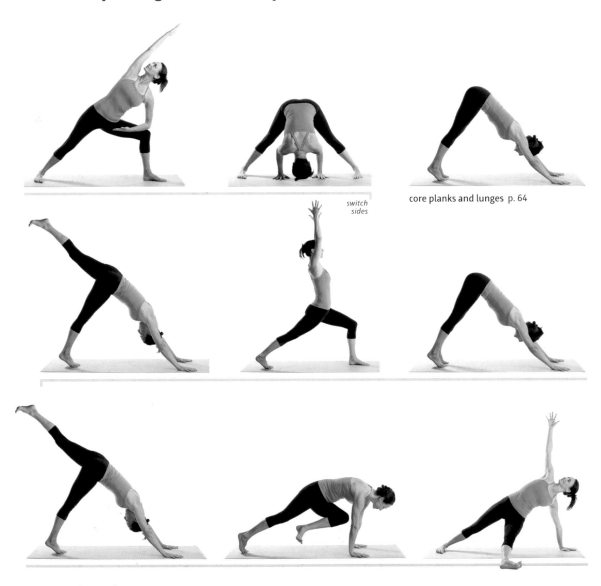

*switch sides*

core planks and lunges  p. 64

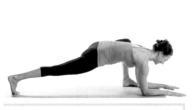

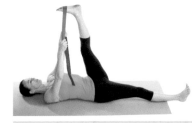

*switch
sides*

strap stretches  p. 78

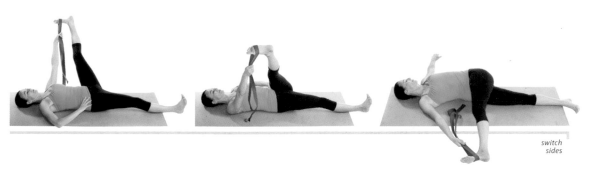

*switch
sides*

# lower-body flexibility and mobility

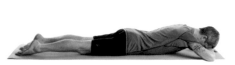

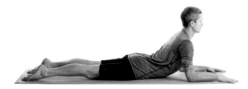

six moves of the spine, prone, bent knee  p. 34

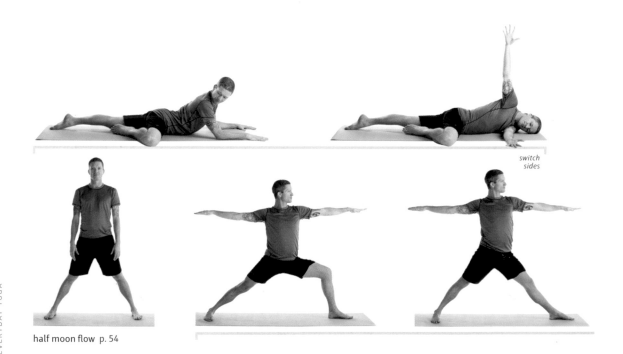

*switch sides*

half moon flow  p. 54

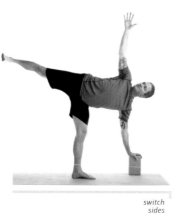

*switch
sides*

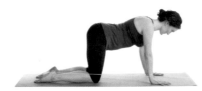

"Christina's World" p. 66

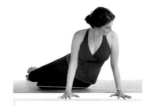

*switch
sides*

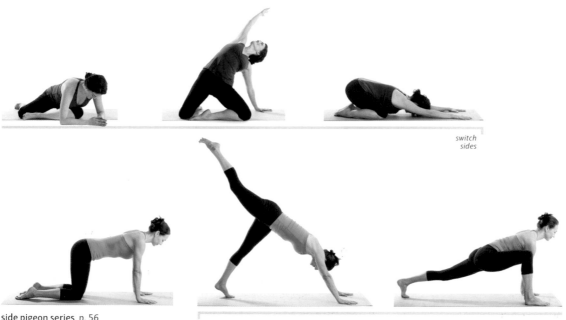

side pigeon series  p. 56

*continued*

# lower-body flexibility and mobility *continued*

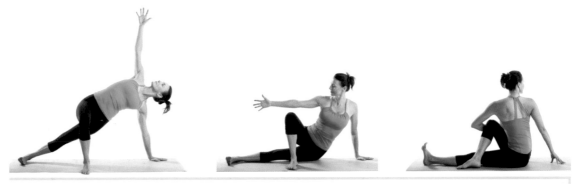

*switch sides*

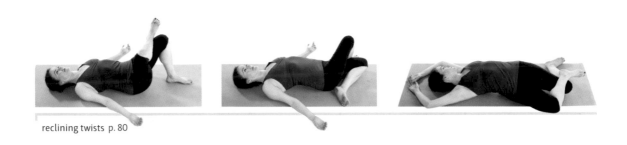

reclining twists p. 80

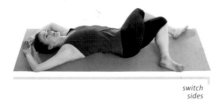

*switch sides*

# upper-body strength and stability

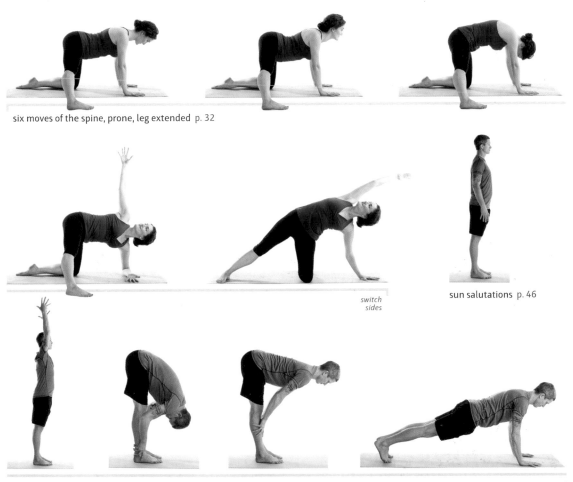

six moves of the spine, prone, leg extended  p. 32

*switch sides*

sun salutations  p. 46

*continued*

# upper-body strength and stability *continued*

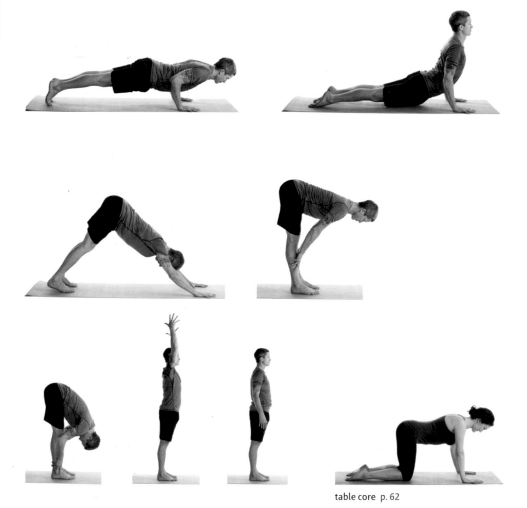

table core p. 62

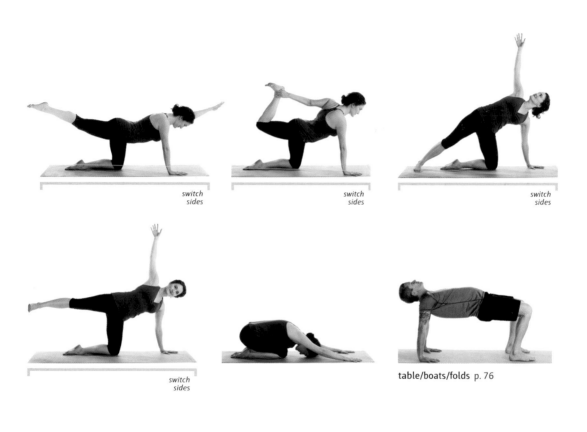

*switch
sides*

*switch
sides*

*switch
sides*

*switch
sides*

table/boats/folds p. 76

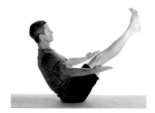

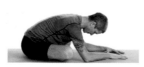

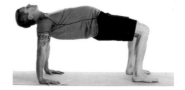

*continued*

# upper-body strength and stability *continued*

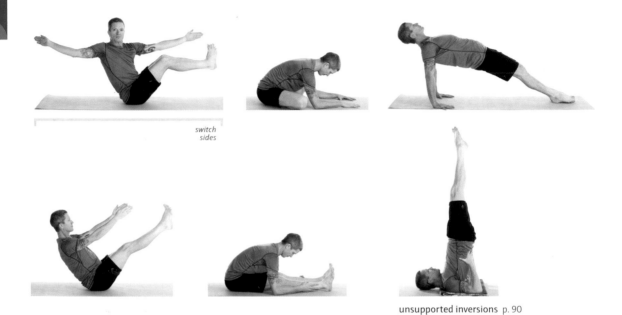

*switch sides*

unsupported inversions  p. 90

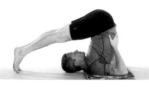
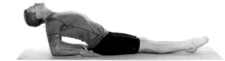

# upper-body flexibility and mobility

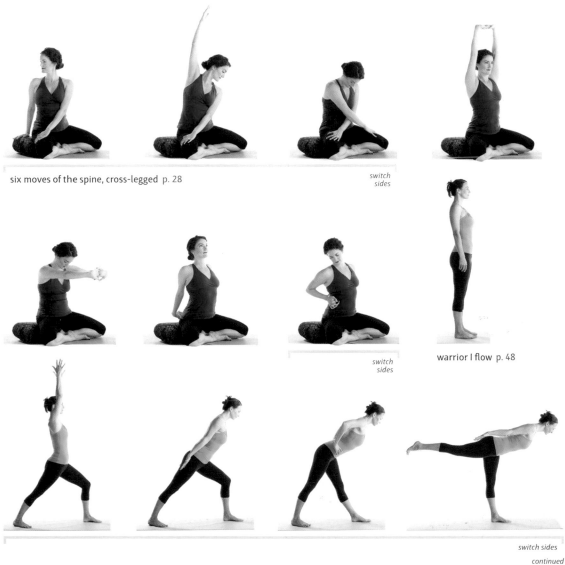

six moves of the spine, cross-legged  p. 28

*switch sides*

*switch sides*

warrior I flow  p. 48

*switch sides*

*continued*

# upper-body flexibility and mobility *continued*

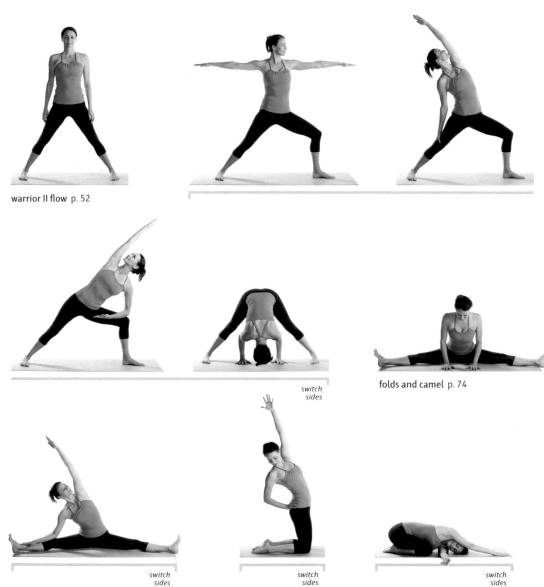

warrior II flow  p. 52

*switch
sides*

folds and camel  p. 74

*switch
sides*

*switch
sides*

*switch
sides*

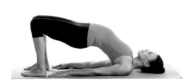
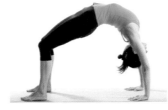
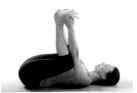

backbends and happy baby   p. 88

# relaxation and recovery

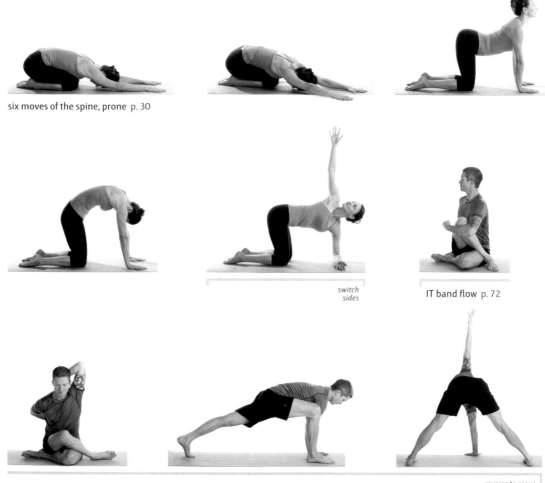

six moves of the spine, prone  p. 30

*switch sides*

IT band flow  p. 72

*reverse to move back to left*

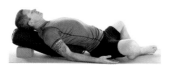

restorative six moves of the spine  p. 96

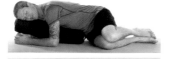

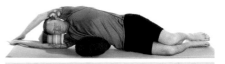

*switch sides*

*switch sides*

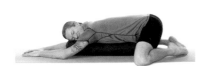

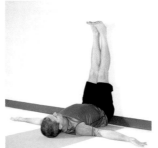

legs up the wall  p. 94

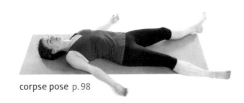

corpse pose p. 98

# organizing your
## everyday
# yoga

The beauty of a menu approach to your home practice is its infinite adjustability. You can arrange and combine routines into a variety of practices to suit your fitness level, aspirations, and mood. This book will help you be creative and joyful in your approach. Here are a few ideas to get you rolling. If you're already practicing yoga, the "Everyday Yoga" schedule will be a good fit and provide creative suggestions for your yoga pantry. If your practice frequency is a few times a week, then start with the "Every-Other-Day Yoga" schedule to establish a foundation and appetite for everyday yoga. If you're an athlete juggling multiple workouts each week, the "Twice-a-Week Yoga" schedule will help you integrate yoga into your workout schedule, especially on easy or recovery days. Season each of these to taste with breath and meditation exercises.

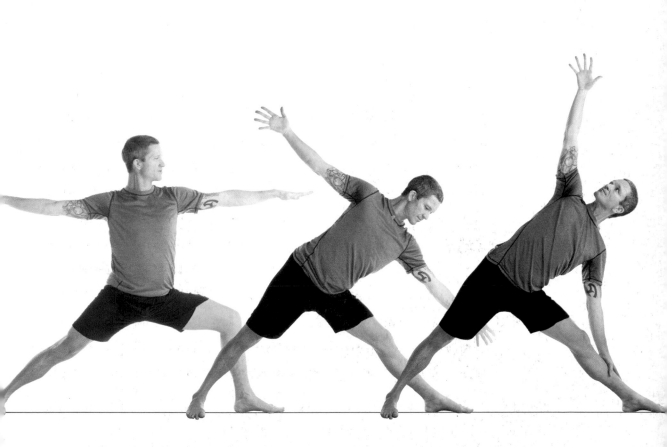

# everyday yoga | Practicing every day gives you the opportunity to meet your body with what it needs, moment to moment. Alternate between short and long practices, and don't hesitate to switch based on how you feel.

## week 1 | sample yoga schedule

| DAY 1 | **Whole-Body Balance** | Six Moves of the Spine, Supine, Two Legs  p. 40 |
| | | Tall Mountain Flow  p. 42 |
| | | Standing Balance Flow  p. 50 |
| | | Dancer/Tree/Pigeon/Eagle  p. 60 |
| | | Head-to-Knee Flow  p. 70 |
| | | Cow-Face/Cobbler  p. 86 |
| DAY 2 | **Upper-Body Strength and Stability** | Six Moves of the Spine, Prone, Leg Extended  p. 32 |
| | | Table Core  p. 62 |
| DAY 3 | **Lower-Body Strength and Stability** | Standing Six Moves of the Spine  p. 24 |
| | | Parking Lot Yoga  p. 44 |
| | | Warrior II Flow  p. 52 |
| | | Core Planks and Lunges  p. 64 |
| | | Strap Stretches  p. 78 |
| DAY 4 | **Core Strength and Stability** | Leg-Swing Flow  p. 36 |
| | | Dynamic Core  p. 68 |
| DAY 5 | **Upper-Body Flexibility and Mobility** | Six Moves of the Spine, Cross-Legged  p. 28 |
| | | Warrior I Flow  p. 48 |
| | | Warrior II Flow  p. 52 |
| | | Folds and Camel  p. 74 |
| | | Backbends and Happy Baby  p. 88 |
| DAY 6 | **Lower-Body Strength and Stability** | Standing Six Moves of the Spine  p. 24 |
| | | Core Planks and Lunges  p. 64 |
| DAY 7 | **Relaxation and Recovery** | Six Moves of the Spine, Prone  p. 30 |
| | | IT Band Flow  p. 72 |
| | | Restorative Six Moves of the Spine  p. 96 |
| | | Legs up the Wall  p. 94 |
| | | Corpse Pose  p. 98 |

## week 2 | sample yoga schedule

| | | | |
|---|---|---|---|
| DAY 1 | **Lower-Body Flexibility and Mobility** | Six Moves of the Spine, Prone, Bent Knee  p. 34<br>Half Moon Flow  p. 54<br>"Christina's World"  p. 66<br>Side Pigeon Series  p. 56<br>Reclining Twists  p. 80 | |
| DAY 2 | **Core Strength and Stability** | Leg-Swing Flow  p. 36<br>Dynamic Core  p. 68 | |
| DAY 3 | **Upper-Body Strength and Stability** | Six Moves of the Spine, Prone, Leg Extended  p. 32<br>Sun Salutations  p. 46<br>Table Core  p. 62<br>Table/Boats/Folds  p. 76<br>Unsupported Inversions  p. 90 | |
| DAY 4 | **Relaxation** | Six Moves of the Spine, Supine, One Leg  p. 38<br>Wall Series  p. 82 | |
| DAY 5 | **Core Strength and Stability** | Leg-Swing Flow  p. 36<br>Planks and Backbends  p. 58<br>Dynamic Core  p. 68<br>Bridge to Block  p. 84<br>Supported Inversions  p. 92 | |
| DAY 6 | **Lower-Body Flexibility and Mobility** | Six Moves of the Spine, Prone, Bent Knee  p. 34<br>Reclining Twists  p. 80 | |
| DAY 7 | **Relaxation and Recovery** | Six Moves of the Spine, Prone  p. 30<br>IT Band Flow  p. 72<br>Restorative Six Moves of the Spine  p. 96 | |

**every-other-day yoga** | Practicing several times a week lets you fit yoga into your days with more flexibility; it also prepares you for most-days or everyday practice.

**week 1** | sample yoga schedule

| | | | |
|---|---|---|---|
| DAY 1 | **Whole-Body Balance** | Six Moves of the Spine, Supine, Two Legs  p. 40<br>Tall Mountain Flow  p. 42<br>Standing Balance Flow  p. 50<br>Dancer/Tree/Pigeon/Eagle  p. 60<br>Head-to-Knee Flow  p. 70<br>Cow-Face/Cobbler  p. 86 | |
| DAY 2 | **Off** | Off | |
| DAY 3 | **Lower-Body Strength and Stability** | Standing Six Moves of the Spine  p. 24<br>Core Planks and Lunges  p. 64 | |
| DAY 4 | **Off** | Off | |
| DAY 5 | **Core Strength and Stability** | Leg-Swing Flow  p. 36<br>Planks and Backbends  p. 58<br>Dynamic Core  p. 68<br>Bridge to Block  p. 84<br>Supported Inversions  p. 92 | |
| DAY 6 | **Off** | Off | |
| DAY 7 | **Relaxation** | Six Moves of the Spine, Supine, One Leg  p. 38<br>Wall Series  p. 82 | |

## week 2 | sample yoga schedule

| DAY 1 | **Upper-Body Strength and Stability** | Six Moves of the Spine, Prone, Leg Extended   p. 32<br>Table Core   p. 62 |
|---|---|---|
| DAY 2 | **Off** | Off |
| DAY 3 | **Lower-Body Strength and Stability** | Standing Six Moves of the Spine   p. 24<br>Parking Lot Yoga   p. 44<br>Warrior II Flow   p. 52<br>Core Planks and Lunges   p. 64<br>Strap Stretches   p. 78 |
| DAY 4 | **Off** | Off |
| DAY 5 | **Lower-Body Flexibility and Mobility** | Six Moves of the Spine, Prone, Bent Knee   p. 34<br>Reclining Twists   p. 80 |
| DAY 6 | **Off** | Off |
| DAY 7 | **Relaxation** | Six Moves of the Spine, Supine, One Leg   p. 38<br>Wall Series   p. 82 |

# twice-a-week yoga | Aim for a minimum of twice-a-week practices, and you'll see yoga's benefits for your body, breath, and mind.

## longer practices | sample yoga schedule

| DAY 1 | **Whole-Body Balance** | Six Moves of the Spine, Supine, Two Legs  p. 40<br>Tall Mountain Flow  p. 42<br>Standing Balance Flow  p. 50<br>Dancer/Tree/Pigeon/Eagle  p. 60<br>Head-to-Knee Flow  p. 70<br>Cow-Face/Cobbler  p. 86 |
|---|---|---|
| DAY 2 | **Off** | Off |
| DAY 3 | **Off** | Off |
| DAY 4 | **Core Strength and Stability** | Leg-Swing Flow  p. 36<br>Planks and Backbends  p. 58<br>Dynamic Core  p. 68<br>Bridge to Block  p. 84<br>Supported Inversions  p. 92 |
| DAY 5 | **Off** | Off |
| DAY 6 | **Off** | Off |
| DAY 7 | **Off** | Off |

## shorter practices | sample yoga schedule

| DAY 1 | **Core Strength and Stability** | Leg-Swing Flow   p. 36<br>Dynamic Core   p. 68 |
|-------|--------------------------------|------------------------------------------------|
| DAY 2 | **Off** | Off |
| DAY 3 | **Off** | Off |
| DAY 4 | **Upper-Body Flexibility and Mobility** | Six Moves of the Spine, Cross-Legged   p. 28<br>Folds and Camel   p. 74 |
| DAY 5 | **Off** | Off |
| DAY 6 | **Off** | Off |
| DAY 7 | **Off** | Off |

# acknowledgments

This book wouldn't be in your hands if it weren't for the thousands of students who have helped me develop this sequencing model for these routines. Thanks to all of you. Special thanks to my yoga teacher training students and teachers' intensive participants for their explicit questions and implicit challenge to make this sequencing model as clear as possible for everyone, teacher and student alike.

Thanks in particular to Wanda and Roy Williams, dedicated students who are a testament to yoga's power to help us feel a little bit better, inclusive of all circumstances, win or lose. You have been wonderful test subjects and muses in the development of these routines. For her kind listening, her constant humoring of my desire to find a food analogy in every situation, and her uplifting energy whether she's my teacher or my student, thanks to Alexandra DeSiato Marano. Your sweet presence makes every experience spicier.

My friends at prAna are always forthcoming and generous with clothing and support of my work: Thank you. Thanks to Hugger Mugger for the props we used in this book.

Thanks to the VeloPress crew: Iris Llewellyn, Casey Blaine, Vicki Hopewell, Dave Trendler, and Connie Oehring; copy editor Jonathan Harrison and proofreader Shena Redmond; the models, Kirsten Warner and Rob Loud; and the photographer, Seth Hughes.

Finally, thanks to my business partner and co-teacher, Lies Sapp, and to my husband, Wes. I love to share meals and linger at the table with you both, and I especially appreciate the way each of you cleans up the kitchen after I've made a mess cooking.

# about the models

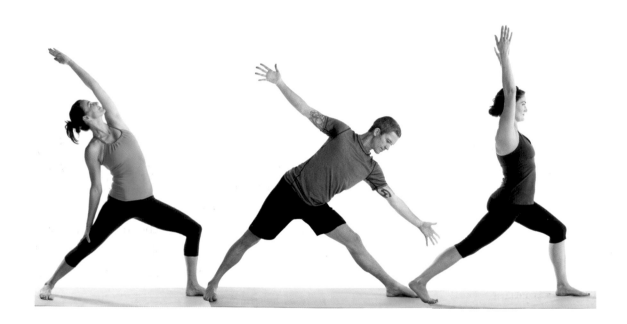

### KIRSTEN WARNER

As a devoted student, heartfelt teacher, and yogini goddess supermom, Kirsten endeavors to live her yoga on and off the mat. She lives in Boulder, Colorado.

www.kirstenwarner.com

### ROB LOUD

Rob is a full-time yoga student and teacher who lives in Boulder, Colorado. He shares his love for yoga practice through every connection.

www.robloudyoga.com

### SAGE ROUNTREE

Sage loves—and loves teaching—a practice that meets the practitioner with both appropriate challenge and plenty of comfort, including an extra-long savasana.

www.sagerountree.com

# about the author

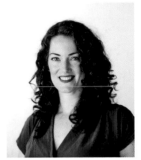

**Sage Rountree's** previous books include *The Athlete's Pocket Guide to Yoga*, *The Runner's Guide to Yoga*, and *Racing Wisely*. With more than a decade of experience teaching yoga, Sage is an experienced registered yoga teacher at the highest level (E-RYT 500) with the Yoga Alliance. Sage is on the faculty of the Kripalu Center for Yoga and Health and teaches yoga classes and yoga teacher trainings internationally and online. She lives with her husband and daughters in Chapel Hill, North Carolina, and co-owns the Carolina Yoga Company, where she heads the 200- and 500-hour yoga teacher training programs.